HOLY & HORMONAL

A FAITH-FILLED GUIDE TO UNDERSTANDING YOUR BODY AND THE GOD WHO DESIGNED YOU

KIM GARGANO

ZONDERVAN BOOKS

ZONDERVAN BOOKS

Holy and Hormonal

Published by Zondervan, 3950 Sparks Drive SE, Suite 101, Grand Rapids, MI 49546, USA. Zondervan is a registered trademark of The Zondervan Corporation, L.L.C., a wholly owned subsidiary of HarperCollins Christian Publishing, Inc.

Requests for information should be addressed to customercare@harpercollins.com.

Zondervan titles may be purchased in bulk for educational, business, fundraising, or sales promotional use. For information, please email SpecialMarkets@Zondervan.com.

ISBN 978-0-310-37038-3 (audio)

Library of Congress Cataloging-in-Publication Data

Names: Gargano, Kim, 1998– author
Title: Holy and hormonal : a faith-filled guide to understanding your body and the God who designed you / Kim Gargano.
Description: Grand Rapids, MI, USA : Zondervan Books, [2026]
Identifiers: LCCN 2026006158 (print) | LCCN 2026006159 (ebook) | ISBN 9780310370345 trade paperback | ISBN 9780310370376 ebook
Subjects: LCSH: Human body—Religious aspects—Christianity | Christian women—Religious life | Menstruation—Religious aspects—Christianity | Menopause—Religious aspects—Christianity
Classification: LCC BT741.3 .G375 2025 (print) | LCC BT741.3 (ebook)
LC record available at https://lccn.loc.gov/2026006158
LC ebook record available at https://lccn.loc.gov/2026006159

The author is represented by Alive Literary Agency, www.aliveliterary.com.

HarperCollins Publishers, Macken House, 39/40 Mayor Street Upper, Dublin 1, D01 C9W8, Ireland (https://www.harpercollins.com)

Cover design: Lindy Kasler
Cover illustrations: Bibadash/Shutterstock
Interior design: Sara Guild

Printed in the United States of America

26 27 28 29 30 LBC 5 4 3 2 1

CONTENTS

INTRODUCTION

I GREW UP IN CENTRAL NEW JERSEY DURING THE ERA OF VICTORIA'S Secret Angels, Juicy Couture tracksuits, low-rise skinny jeans, dark eyeliner in the waterline, and side bags (late '90s babies, if you know you know). The schools I attended shaped me with a strict, disciplined environment where the expectation was clear: keep quiet, listen, and obey. I struggled with being bullied, making friends, and making sense of God and the world around me. As a curious, sensitive kid raised in a culture that kept things hush-hush, I quickly learned that questions and opinions were not welcome. By the time I hit puberty, I had created a cozy, safe space for my feelings: It was a little corner of my brain where I'd retreat to, a place where nobody could hurt me and where I could be free.

Topics like women's health, periods, and mental health were taboo at the time. Menstrual health was *not* a topic of conversation in my family. It was brushed over, pushed aside, and tabled for a different day. But to be fair, the women in my family also lacked women they could turn to for answers. Generations and generations of women have learned to hide the very parts of themselves that make them beautiful creations of God.

As my body developed, the more out of control I felt with what was happening "down there." I'd be doubled over on the bathroom floor with cramps, gripped by irritability that came out of nowhere, and swept up in emotional outbursts I couldn't understand. "Welcome to womanhood!" kept ringing in my ears.

This loneliness continued into my adult life—until quite recently. One simple moment in a parking lot changed my story.

In the thick of my luteal phase (more on this later), I was dealing with some of the worst premenstrual dysphoric disorder (PMDD) symptoms I'd had in a while (more on that later too). My body and mind felt riddled with extreme mood swings, sudden bursts of anger, crying spells, anxiety, and an overall feeling of being "on edge." Sitting in my parked car trying not to punch the steering wheel, I took to YouTube to try to find another woman of faith to encourage me. I typed "periods, hormones, Jesus" into the search bar, and to my surprise, not a single video appeared. It was shocking that nobody seemed to have preached a sermon or given a talk on this, like, ever. Obviously, this discovery added to my frustration, and I started to sob in my Honda Civic. *I must be going crazy.*

After my emotional outburst, I felt the Lord prompt me to film a video discussing those very frustrations. Social media has always been an outlet for me, so I propped up my phone and began my rant.

"Guys, I think I'm going insane! I love Jesus with my

whole heart, but I do not have any faith today. My period is hitting me like a truck. Please tell me I'm not alone in this."

Pressing "Post," I didn't think anything of it for the next few hours.

When I opened TikTok later that day, I was overwhelmed with the amount of support and love I had received. To my surprise, the video went viral and over two million women from around the world shared similar experiences in the comment section. Women said that they were grateful someone finally had started talking about faith and our hormones, and some expressed that they had never felt more seen and validated.

That encouragement was a powerful reminder that I wasn't in this alone. Every month, I was cycling in solidarity with women all over the globe, going through the hormonal ups and downs that are part of my female identity—a common experience to celebrate and share, not one to hide or feel ashamed of. It connected me to a larger community, reminding me of the strength and resilience that comes from embracing who we are as beloved daughters of Christ.

The more I learned, the more I realized that this connection doesn't disappear as we age—it deepens, expanding into new seasons and new shared experiences. It has been truly incredible to witness the unwavering flood of support for the new menopause awareness movement. After years of being pushed into the shadows, women are finally stepping into the light with confidence, boldly embracing their bodies, and demanding the care and attention they've been denied for far too long. From a faith perspective, this unity is a powerful reminder of what can happen when women come together as the body of Christ—when we are seen, heard, and understood by God and by one another. It's a testimony to the strength we gain when we stand together and lift each other up, no matter what age we are.

Even so, the struggle continues. The women who responded to my video were decrying a Western culture that still doesn't know how to handle the reality of women's bodies. Unrealistic beauty standards, misogynistic ideologies, and a lack of scientific research in women's health have all contributed to our continuing nervousness about our bodies and the blood that comes out of them.

Historically, before the 1990s women were rarely included in clinical research. In 1993 the National Institutes of Health (NIH) Revitalization Act mandated the inclusion of women in all NIH-funded clinical research, marking a turning point in women's history.[1] Though it's a step in the right direction and the number of female participants is rising, it isn't perfect, and women are still significantly underrepresented.

A 2021 cross-sectional analysis of clinical trials from 2007 to 2020 found that obstetrical complications affect more than a third of women globally, yet only 2 percent of all clinical trials in the US are obstetrical.[2] But that imbalance isn't only in the participants; as of 2023 women lead roughly 32 percent of clinical trials, while men lead 64 percent.[3] It saddens my heart to know that although women account for half the population, we're not treated as equals.

Women are not little men. We're our own gender, with different hormonal profiles, different responses to everyday stress, and a different biological makeup. On average, women operate on a twenty-eight-day hormonal cycle, whereas men operate on a twenty-four-hour cycle. This means it takes women twenty-eight days to move through all the hormones, emotions, and flavors of humanhood. While men can wake up feeling the same every day, some women wake up not knowing what version of themselves they're going to get. Simply put, women primarily produce the hormones estrogen and progesterone, which regulate reproductive cycles and regulate many of our female traits. Men primarily produce testosterone, influencing bone density, muscle mass, and the functioning of the male reproductive system.

When it comes to things like stress, men typically jump into fight-or-flight mode. Women sometimes do that too, but we also have a tend-and-befriend response thanks to higher estrogen and oxytocin levels. Instead of pulling away, we're wired to seek connection, comfort, or protection for others—basically, we go into mama-bear mode while men either charge ahead or check out.

Women have had the instinct to nurture and protect for thousands of years, shaping not only how we respond to stressors but also how we've been perceived by society. Our periods have been especially political. These challenges aren't unique to today—they go back to the early church and beyond. If you've ever read Leviticus, you've seen words like *unclean* used to describe menstruation: "Whenever a woman has her menstrual period, she will be ceremonially unclean for seven days. Anyone who touches her during that time will be unclean until evening. Anything on which the woman lies or sits during the time of her period will be unclean" (Leviticus 15:19–20 NLT).

I know, I know. I had the same initial reaction you're having right now: *Jeez. That's aggressive.* Keep reading until verse 30; it'll make you grateful for Jesus!

It's hard to read out-of-context verses like these and believe God's design for our bodies is wonderful and miraculous. It's even harder to celebrate our bodies when we've been told for centuries that we're dirty ogres who need to be separated from society so our cooties don't get on anything.

But you are an image bearer of the Lord Himself, so if someone has something to say about you, tell them to take it up with God.

Throughout this journey, you and I will take a closer look at verses like this to truly understand what the Lord's heart is for His daughters. We will work together to understand the cultural and historical context we live in. And most importantly, we will reclaim the beauty of womanhood and fall in love with God's design for us.

That has been my biggest prayer with this book, with my podcast, and with this ministry: that women feel less alone, less crazy, and a little more in love with their body and the One who created it. I've read countless books on periods, sifted through endless research articles, listened to hormone health experts speak on podcasts and in seminars, and even spoken on a few podcasts myself. But the one thing I found missing from all the literature and conversations was Jesus. Reading book after book, I wanted to scream into the pages, "God is everywhere in this! Why aren't we crediting Him?" It became my mission to bridge the gap between faith and science. I took it so far that I got my certification as an integrative nutritionist and hormone health coach. This mission is my passion and the very reason God put me here on this earth.

My greatest desire is for women of all ages and walks of life to find comfort and belonging here. From the twelve-year-old girl who is discovering her body for the first time, to the college student who can't get a grip on her hormonal imbalances, to the married woman struggling to conceive, to the woman suffering the loss of a baby. From the woman struggling with postpartum depression to the woman entering menopause. Whether you're single, dating, engaged, married, divorced, widowed, or have your relationship status set to "Over. It." I wrote this book for you.

For the structure of this book, I wanted the sections and chapters to mimic the roller coaster we often ride while going through our menstrual cycle (and everyday life too). It often starts with a feeling and an expression of that feeling, good or bad. Then that feeling turns into questioning: Why *do* I feel this way? What's going on inside my mind and body that's causing this feeling or reaction? How can I understand what's happening so I have more control over the outcome? Once we have that understanding, we act. We set goals, come up with a plan, figure out ways to prevent a certain behavior, find new routines, and set ourselves up for success.

The flow of this book will imitate that pattern. We'll spend a lot of time relating to each other by opening the floor for long-overdue conversations about our periods. Together, we'll take a sigh of relief and hold space for validation and healing. We'll cry about our past experiences, grieve the younger versions of ourselves that deserved better, and invite the Holy Spirit to step in and speak a better word over us. Then we'll journey into the beautiful, complex, and divine biology of the female body. We will dive into the science of our menstrual cycle, understand and identify hormonal imbalances, and discover the woman God created you to be in all your unique individuality. We'll cry together as you read the honest, tender stories of brave women who have walked through miscarriage, infertility, and heartbreaking loss yet were willing to open their hearts so you wouldn't feel alone. You'll even hear from the doctor who delivered me from my mother's womb as he answers commonly asked questions about fertility and discusses how he sees God everywhere in his line of work.

And finally, you will learn practical tools and tips to live in harmony with your body. You'll learn to go with your flow (literally) and allow the Lord to lead you through each phase of your cycle. We'll do a deep dive into cycle syncing, break stereotypes and false narratives about worship, learn how to armor up spiritually amid shifting hormones, and most importantly, find a healthy balance between faith and feelings.

I want you to know I'm so proud of you. Your journey is not easy. Being a woman is not easy. We've been neglected emotionally, physically, and spiritually by others and even by ourselves. Satan has perverted what being a woman means by feeding us lies, creating anxiety and insecurity, and pushing a false identity down our throats—one that tells us we're defined by the world's opinions instead of God's truth about us.

Enough is enough. It's time to link arms and charge forward as the Lord parts the red sea (pun intended). We're suiting up with the armor of God while standing firm on the truth of who we are. We're daughters of the King! It's time for the world to see women walking securely in their true identity, living in freedom with their bodies, and being confident in the calling God established for them.

As Psalm 139:14 says,

> I praise you because I am fearfully and
> wonderfully made;
> your works are wonderful,
> I know that full well.

You're fearfully and wonderfully made. It's time to start believing it.

PART ONE

THE PERIOD TALK YOU NEVER HAD

ONE

IT'S NOT YOUR FAULT YOU DIDN'T KNOW

PICTURE THIS: A TWELVE-YEAR-OLD GIRL ON A FAMILY VACATION at the beach, wearing a bikini with a tampon string hanging out of the bottoms. An embarrassing callout is followed by a family member's pointing and laughing. A chorus of giggles and whispers. Flushed cheeks. Humiliation. A lump in her throat. She panics and makes a beeline for the nearest bathroom. She's filled with a crushing sense of shame.

You guessed it—that girl was me. I vividly remember that day because it deeply scarred me. Still new to my period, I hadn't yet figured out how to insert a tampon properly. No female figure in my life tried to explain how it works. So there I was, with shaky hands and a racing heart, unfolding from the tampon box what looked like a mile-long accordion of gibberish. The print was so small it would've taken me hours to get to step one, and by that time the sun would have set and my beach time would be over. *Who reads those things anyway?*

I tossed the paper aside and decided to wing it. How hard could it be, right? You just put it inside and, bam, done. Nope! Boy, was I wrong! Instead of inserting the applicator, I pushed the cotton up, threw the applicator aside, and shoved the dry, hard cotton as far inside me as I could. Despite the pain, I kept maneuvering it to a point where I assumed it should sit. "This is my rite of passage to womanhood, right? Better get used to the pain and discomfort now." Pulling up my shorts, I noticed an unpleasant sensation and pressure down there. "Whatever," I thought, "this is normal." I winced every step I took from the house to the beach.

"How are the girls in the Playtex commercials doing cartwheels, running five-hundred-meter sprints, and competing in tennis tournaments? What the heck am I missing?"

Moseying down the beach to where my family had set up camp, I spotted a family member in the water with a handful of other women I didn't know. Removing my shorts and tank top, I headed for the water to join the group. She shot me a look of confusion, as if she was trying to figure out what was out of order with me.

Pointing at my bottoms, she shouted, "Is that a tampon string?!" Hysterical laughter erupted, along with a choir of giggles and looks of agreement among the strangers. Mortified, I looked down and saw the string hanging out of my bikini. Heat rushed to my face, my throat swelled, and my eyes welled up with tears. To say I was humiliated would be an understatement. I had already felt insecure because I was forced to figure out how to use a tampon on my own, and now I had a group of women who should have supported me but instead used me as the object of their entertainment.

Desperately throwing my shorts back on, I ran for the nearest bathroom and cried as I yanked the tampon out of my body. A crushing sense of shame washed over me. I was alone, embarrassed, defeated, and in physical pain.

From a very young age I was left to figure out a lot of things on my own. I was a twelve-year-old girl desperate for guidance and support but had never felt more embarrassed and ashamed. I learned to internalize my feelings and associate periods with things to be kept hidden. And while my mom did the best she could with what she knew, neither of us had the tools or language to navigate this season well. So I withdrew into myself and became isolated in my feelings and raging hormones.

By the time high school hit, my periods were dreadful. My flow was incredibly heavy, and my mood swings were terrible. One minute I was happy, the next I was depressed. One minute I was friendly and social, the next I needed to be alone and silent. One minute I felt peaceful, the next I wanted to kick someone in the face. One moment I was smiling at my neighbor, the next I wanted to light their house on fire. It felt like my body was playing tug-of-war with me and I was losing no matter which side I leaned toward. Keeping up with sports, friends, and grades was already stressful, and with my period thrown into the mix, it was an uphill battle. Because my mood swings were drastic, my attitude and behaviors were unpredictable. I struggled to maintain friendships due to my moodiness and inconsistency. Premenstrual syndrome (PMS) would turn my sensitive, empathetic self into a judgmental, apathetic, and unapologetic person. When my period was about to start, I no longer recognized who I was. It was as if my tender heart and caring nature went out the door and the queen of doom entered the room. And the kicker was, I couldn't control it! I had no tools to flip the script: I was constantly at the mercy of my hormones.

Is this just my experience, or is it yours too? Can you recall a time when you felt embarrassed or ashamed of your period? Have you ever hidden a tampon up your sleeve when going to the bathroom in a restaurant? Or have you silenced the sound of breaking open a pad with the loud whoosh of a flushed toilet? Do you feel uncomfortable talking to other women about periods? If you answered yes to any of these questions, you're not alone. For decades women's health has been brushed off, cast aside, and set on the back burner. Women have suffered in silence, bearing the emotional and physical load in isolation. This chasm has separated women not only from medical practitioners but also from each other.

Three key factors have contributed to women feeling misunderstood or uninformed about their own bodies—specifically about their menstrual cycles: lack of scientific research, misogynistic ideologies, and unrealistic beauty standards. These factors have not only created a void of knowledge but also fostered an environment where women feel isolated or ashamed of a natural and essential part of their lives.

LACK OF SCIENTIFIC RESEARCH

As noted previously, women were rarely included in clinical research study until the 1993 National Institutes of Health Revitalization Act, which mandated the inclusion of women and minorities in all NIH-funded clinical research. But let's back it up a few years to understand why this ban even came into effect. From the 1930s to the 1970s, devastatingly unethical and immoral human experimentation for medical research was done on African American men diagnosed with late latent syphilis—a sexually transmitted infection—in Tuskegee, Alabama. The purpose of the study was to follow the natural history of untreated syphilis in African American men twenty-five years or older. All the men were informed that they were taking part in a study, but they were not properly educated about its implications. The study was unethical for many reasons, the first being that researchers did not adhere to the scientific standards of ethical conduct, in part by not receiving informed consent from the participants. The second reason was that the men were not offered treatment, even after it was readily available during the penicillin boom.[1] Basically, these men were left untreated of syphilis as a part of a medical study. The public outcry sparked the National Research Act of 1974, a piece of legislation establishing a system to oversee and regulate human experimentation in research to ensure ethical, safe practices and to protect the participants.

Shortly after, the 1977 FDA guidance recommended excluding women of "childbearing age" from participating in Phases I and II of drug trials due to the risks of new therapies and treatments.[2] From the 1970s to '90s, medical technologies greatly advanced. Unfortunately, the unintended side effect of excluding women meant that most of the research we have today is from procedures, medications, and imaging tools tested on men. Remember how I said women are not tiny men? This male-centric approach to research has had long-lasting consequences for women.

Here are some discrepancies between men and women in cardiology according to Northwell Health:

- Women are more likely to die after a heart attack than men.
- Heart attack symptoms look very different in men (crushing chest pain) than in women (nausea, fatigue, shortness of breath). Though these differences are known, doctors are still trained to look for male heart attack symptoms.
- Standard treatments, such as angioplasty and stents, were designed with men in mind. Uncoincidentally, women are more likely than men to have adverse cardiovascular events after the placement of a stent.[3]

While the gender gap in medical research has gained attention in recent years, the gynecological and reproductive health fields still face significant disparities. In clinical trials, women of childbearing age are not well represented in studies for drugs or treatments related to their health needs because medical professionals fear fertility damage or assume that women's bodies will respond the same as men's. Another reason may be a presumption that women's hormones are too unpredictable in the childbearing years. As you'll learn by the end of this book, the menstrual cycle is one of the most reliable and predictable functions of the body, so we can debunk that belief right now.

We've come a long way since 1993 but still have quite a way to go. According to the Endometriosis Foundation of America, it takes women an average of ten years to receive an endometriosis diagnosis.[4] For polycystic ovary syndrome (PCOS), it takes two to three years.[5] I can't imagine the years of pain and the countless unanswered questions that women have endured, often for decades, before finally receiving an accurate diagnosis. This injustice must change, and I believe God positioned this generation to be the catalyst for that transformation. As women begin to demand equal treatment in medicine, we stand in prayer, trusting that lasting change will unfold. Every woman deserves the validation and care that has too long been denied, and together, in Jesus's name, we will ensure they receive it.

MISOGYNISTIC IDEOLOGIES

The second contributor to our lack of information and feeling of isolation is misogynistic ideologies—the faulty beliefs that women are inferior to men, should be subjugated, and are less deserving of the same rights, respect, and opportunities. These ideologies have been embedded in history through culture, religion, and social structures. A few examples include economic inequality for women, the sexualization and objectification of the female body, discrimination against women in healthcare, and gender stereotypes of women. As much as we want to believe that this way of thinking is in the past, it very much exists today.

How many times have you been catcalled walking down the street? Or manipulated into doing a sexual act? Can you recall a time when you had to fight tooth and nail for a pay raise while your male coworker was getting handed bonuses on a silver platter? Has a man ever told you that you belong in the kitchen? Or maybe you overheard a group of men degrading women all in the name of a "joke." The term used to describe these frat bro characteristics is *toxic masculinity*. It's every woman's worst nightmare in a man: emotional unavailability, a need for dominance and control, and a "men don't cry" toughness. It's the opposite of Jesus and the characteristics He displayed while on earth.

A lot of these toxic traits are learned behaviors passed from father to son. Some little boys grow up with an emotionally distant dad who never shows them affection or celebrates their wins, and they process this coldness as normal behavior. Or maybe they see the way Dad speaks to Mom: stern, demanding, and apathetic. Maybe they witnessed their mom in pain or discomfort because of her period, and instead of their dad stepping in to offer support, he made a passing comment that period blood is gross and she was just being dramatic. Maybe the belittling focused on her body, her outward appearance, or her pain—cementing in their minds that women's value is conditional. In any case, this type of rhetoric makes women seem small and unworthy and men seem powerful and in control.

Religion and culture have also played a part in fueling the male-centric fire. During the time Jesus lived on earth, women were looked down on. They had few, if any, rights and no credibility. But Jesus is pro-women. Hallelujah! The first people He revealed Himself to after the resurrection were two women: Mary Magdalene and Mary the mother of James and Joseph. A woman's testimony was generally not legally valid in that era, so it's incredible that Jesus flipped the script and chose women to relay the good news of our resurrected King.

Breaking free from the chains of misogynistic ideologies requires a deep shift and intentional change in how we see women and empower them to love the bodies God gave them.

UNREALISTIC BEAUTY STANDARDS

Women have long dealt with unrealistic beauty standards, like weighing a certain amount and having flawless skin, straight white teeth, a thin waist, and a certain texture hair—the list is never-ending and always changing. In addition, I want to call attention to the perfectionism women wrestle with and the fear of failure or embarrassment that keeps women chained. In my own life, the fear of not looking perfect, acting perfectly, speaking perfectly, or finishing a job perfectly created anxiety and shame within me. Maybe you can relate to this feeling in your own way, whether that's beating yourself up for falling short on a presentation at work or wearing oversized clothing to hide your body. We all have insecurities, but the sad reality is that our bodies were never supposed to become objects of shame. Other people's self-made standards have dimmed the light that God intended to shine brightly.

Another huge problem I see in this generation (and within myself) is the comparison and insecurity that arise because of social media use. JAMA Network performed a study on fifty-three thousand teens and looked at how time spent on their phones affected how they saw their bodies. They found that teens who used their phones for more than five hours a day were more likely to see their bodies inaccurately, often thinking they were heavier than they really were and resorting to unhealthy methods to lose weight.[6] The moral of the story is this: The more time you spend comparing yourself with others, the more you forget how loved and valued you are by God. This is why Paul says in Romans 12:2, "Do not conform to the pattern of this world, but be transformed by the renewing of your mind. Then you will be able to test and approve what God's will is—his good, pleasing and perfect will."

God doesn't want us to look at other people for validation and worth. He knows the pain and heartbreak that come from doing that, which is why He instructs us to be transformed into a new person—one who looks to *Him* for identity and worth. The next time you catch yourself comparing or wishing you looked like someone else, pause and remember: You are already loved and chosen. The world tells you to edit, filter, and perform to be good enough. God says you already are.

REDEFINING WHAT IT MEANS TO BE "UNCLEAN"

Part of breaking the cycle of misogyny is facing the uncomfortable facts about where some of these beliefs and attitudes began. To do that, let's go back to the ancient laws and cultural views that shaped how women—and their menstrual cycles—were perceived. The law of Moses states that women are unclean during their periods. Numbers 5:2 says, "Command the Israelites to send away from the camp anyone who has a defiling skin disease or a discharge of any kind [this includes women on their periods], or who is ceremonially unclean because of a dead body." Leviticus 15:19–20 (NLT) echoes the same point: "Whenever a woman has her menstrual period, she will be ceremonially unclean for seven days. Anyone who touches her during that time will be unclean until evening. Anything on which the woman lies or sits during the time of her period will be unclean." That's difficult to read, isn't it? Those considered unclean were separated from God's presence and their community. They were sent to the outskirts of town and could return to fellowship with God's people only after waiting their allotted time, undergoing a cleansing ritual, and offering a sacrifice.

Where is God in all of this? How could our periods possibly be worth celebrating? Does He see women as gross and unclean?

From Genesis 3 to the present day, we see the consequences of Eve's actions unfolding: pain and suffering.

There's a running theme in the Bible of women in pain, from Hagar and Naomi to the woman with the issue of blood in the New Testament. Emotional and physical pain are not foreign experiences for us. It seems unfair, but there's a beautiful story here that points straight to Jesus and His redemption.

Jesus is the ultimate sacrifice, and through His blood that was shed, He brought forth new life. Like our cycles, and much like birth, it was the shedding of blood for the bringing of new life. Who can better relate to us than the One who bled for you and me? God humbled Himself to be born in a stable, screaming and covered in blood from a woman's body. He would go on to heal women and girls, never afraid of becoming unclean by their touch, but healing them physically, emotionally, and spiritually.

Hebrews 13:11–13 perfectly captures the beauty, awesomeness, and grace of Jesus: "The high priest carries the blood of animals into the Most Holy Place as a sin offering, but the bodies are burned outside the camp. And so Jesus also suffered outside the city gate to make the people holy through his own blood. Let us, then, go to him outside the camp, bearing the disgrace he bore." Jesus not only saw our pain but took it upon Himself and joined us in it—so when we retreat to the lonely corners, the isolated spaces, or the places we think no one else would ever follow, we find Him already there, waiting to restore us.

Here's an invitation to see your menstrual cycle in a different light: as a representation of God's selfless, redeeming love. In fact, God redefines the world's perception of love and cleanliness. While the world defines our period as gross and unclean, God sees it as a sacred, divine reflection of His grace, power, and healing. And let's not forget that one of Jesus's favorite things is rest. Though the ancient Israelite women were sent to the outskirts, they were invited to rest. They were given a space to be joined in community, encouraging and supporting one another in their discomfort. How kind of the Father not only to prepare a place for them to decompress but to be there with us, ministering to us in our most vulnerable moments too.

The ways you've been neglected and the pain you feel are valid. There's a lot we're up against—from the unnecessary opinions of others, to toxic ideologies about women, to the lack of representation in the medical field. The road to change can feel like walking up a downward escalator. Over the years I've received many messages from women expressing their deep frustration, hopelessness, and even grief over how their bodies have been misunderstood or dismissed. I've sat with women at the end of their rope and held their pain with them. Some have carried these wounds for decades, and others are just now finding the language to describe what they've been through. But together, with Jesus at the center, we can be the ones to say enough is enough. Jesus's love is the catalyst for change—the love of "the God who sees me," as Hagar named the Lord in her deepest pain (Genesis 16:13).

Through Him we stand tall with our shoulders back, confident in our true identity as beloved daughters of Christ.

PRACTICAL APPLICATION

- The next time you're at the OB/GYN, speak up for yourself and ask questions.
- Try opening up to a friend or family member about your hardships and see what happens. You can go into it guarding your heart, but let the walls down if there's an opportunity for connection.
- Ask the Lord if there are any people in your life you need to forgive.
- Reframe your perspective on your menstrual cycle, seeing it as an invitation to rest rather than a source of shame.

SCRIPTURE TO MEDITATE ON

- "Do not conform to the pattern of this world, but be transformed by the renewing of your mind. Then you will be able to test and approve what God's will is—his good, pleasing and perfect will." (Romans 12:2)
- "The high priest carries the blood of animals into the Most Holy Place as a sin offering, but the bodies are burned outside the camp. And so Jesus also suffered outside the city gate to make the people holy through his own blood. Let us, then, go to him outside the camp, bearing the disgrace he bore." (Hebrews 13:11–13)

TWO

THE FOUR SEASONS OF YOUR CYCLE

HAVE YOU EVER NOTICED THAT YOUR BODY FEELS DIFFERENT WEEK to week? Like some days you're bursting with energy, and others you're craving stillness? That's not by happenstance—it's how God designed the female body. Just as the Lord designed the seasons to move from fall to winter, winter to spring, spring to summer, and summer to fall again, our bodies follow a similar cyclical pattern. In fact, many things follow a cycle. The sun rises and sets; the moon goes through a 29.5-day cycle; the tides rise and fall; trees in the forest grow, mature, and eventually die, falling to the ground to decompose and provide nutrients for new growth. We too have biological cycles. The menstrual cycle is more than bleeding and then not bleeding—it's a four-phase hormonal symphony, mirroring the very seasons we see in creation.

As women, we have a menstrual cycle. Everybody is different, but for the sake of averages, a young woman's first period (menarche) occurs between twelve and thirteen years of age,[1] with an average cycle length of twenty-eight days (though twenty-one to thirty-five days is considered a normal, healthy range).[2] During these twenty-eight days, our bodies move through a variety of hormonal fluctuations, affecting energy, motivation, strength, appetite, sleep quality, metabolism, reproduction, mental focus, creativity, ability to handle stress, and weight. Should I keep going? Our menstrual cycle affects every aspect of our lives. It's deeply complex, wildly underestimated, and one hundred percent the cornerstone of womanhood. So much so that the American College of Obstetricians and Gynecologists introduced the idea that the menstrual cycle could be considered the "fifth vital sign," alongside traditional vital signs like heart rate, blood pressure, respiration rate, and temperature.[3] That's how important our periods are when it comes to overall wellness!

The menstrual cycle has four phases: menstrual, follicular, ovulatory, and luteal. These also overlap and can be grouped in two, the first half of your cycle (follicular) and the second half (luteal). If this is news to you, don't worry, you're not alone. I didn't discover this until my early twenties. I know it might seem a bit confusing at first, but bear with me. I'm going to break down each phase in the simplest way possible so you'll one day be able to explain it clearly to your friends and family.

Before we jump into each phase and season, allow me to introduce you to your new besties, three of the most important hormones for menstrual health.

Ready?

Introducing the "hype girl," a.k.a. estrogen. Estrogen is a powerhouse hormone that plays a key role in women's reproductive health. It is produced mainly by the ovaries but also by the adrenal glands (glands responsible for releasing adrenaline and cortisol) and fat cells. Estrogen helps regulate the menstrual cycle and is involved in the development of secondary sexual characteristics like the growth of breasts and widening of hips. It also plays a role in bone health, keeping them strong, and protects against heart disease. Estrogen contributes to confidence, creativity, social stamina, and energy. Think of her as your personal hype girl. She's there to keep you feeling your best so you can tackle any task with boldness and grace! She makes you strong and empowers you to push yourself to reach your full potential.

Next up is the "chill girl," progesterone. Equally as important as her sister estrogen, progesterone is the one to encourage you to slow down, turn inward, and pump the brakes on life. She's self-aware and values boundaries and alone time. Progesterone is another key hormone produced by the ovaries, specifically the corpus luteum—the structure that forms after an egg is released during ovulation. It helps prepare your body for a potential pregnancy, making the uterine lining thick and nutritient-rich. During pregnancy, progesterone also helps prepare the breasts for milk production. She's the chill girl for a reason, counteracting her rambunctious sister by bringing hormones back into balance, especially in the mind. She calms the uterus by reducing muscle contractions, so if you experience cramps, phone your bestie progesterone to come to the rescue.

And lastly, we have testosterone, the "spicy girl." She loves to get into the nitty-gritty. She may not take the spotlight every day, but when she shows up, things are going to get done. She gives you extra strength in the gym, provides the confidence to speak up, and helps you feel radiant in your own skin. Testosterone is also what contributes to an increase in sex drive, especially during the ovulatory phase. She's a tricky girl sometimes, though, because when she's not at balanced levels, things like acne, low energy, and a lack of focus can arise. She's not a flashy girl like estrogen, but she'll be the one to send you an encouraging text: "Let's do it!"

The four phases are widely recognized as parallels to the four seasons: winter, spring, summer, and fall. As Ecclesiastes 3:1–8 says, for *everything* there is a season. It reads:

> There is a time for everything,
> and a season for every activity under the heavens:
>
> a time to be born and a time to die,
> a time to plant and a time to uproot,
> a time to kill and a time to heal,
> a time to tear down and a time to build,
> a time to weep and a time to laugh,
> a time to mourn and a time to dance,
> a time to scatter stones and a time to gather them,
> a time to embrace and a time to refrain from embracing,

a time to search and a time to give up,
a time to keep and a time to throw away,
a time to tear and a time to mend,
a time to be silent and a time to speak,
a time to love and a time to hate,
a time for war and a time for peace.

Just as creation moves through seasons of rest, growth, blooming, and release, so do our bodies. We reflect God's craftmanship and the holy rhythms He designed. Learning to honor these rhythms rather than fight against them allows us to step into alignment with His perfect timing. In the stillness of winter (menstrual phase), the fresh energy of spring (follicular phase), the fullness of summer (ovulatory phase), and the gentle slowing of fall (luteal phase), we can see His hand at work. Now let's embark on a journey through the four phases to see how the three sisters of estrogen, progesterone, and testosterone come together to make the divine happen!

MENSTRUAL PHASE (WINTER: A TIME FOR PEACE)

Let's start at day 1 of your cycle, which is the beginning of the menstrual phase. This phase begins on the day you start bleeding and lasts anywhere from three to seven days (remember, every woman is different). During this time, your body sheds the uterine lining (the endometrium) it built up in previous phases to prepare your body for a potential pregnancy. This lining is where a fertilized egg would implant if conception occurred. If you're not pregnant, your body gets rid of this lining, and it is expelled through the vagina as blood.

Estrogen and progesterone are wiped out in this phase. In fact, all your sex hormones are at their lowest. They've worked hard to build up your body for pregnancy, and now it's their time to rest. Because your body exerts a ton of energy to shed the uterine lining, you may experience fatigue, exhaustion, inflammation, or weight gain. The endocrine system, which is the body's network of glands and organs that make hormones, is extremely sensitive and doesn't always respond well to these fluctuations, further contributing to things like low energy or even anxiety. Plus, your uterus contracts to get rid of the blood, so it's no wonder you may feel crummy.

These more severe symptoms typically happen during the first few days of your period, but toward the end of your bleed, around day 5, estrogen slowly "wakes up" from her slumber and prepares your body for the next phase. It's almost like the first signs of spring peeking through the snow—renewal is coming.

The menstrual phase is the body's "winter," a time for peace. It's a time to slow down, cozy up on the couch, reflect, and allow yourself to rest. Think of it as a prolonged sabbath, a time God designed for you to pause and recalibrate. Just as the earth rests under a blanket of snow before blooming again, your body requires stillness and nourishment before it can build up strength for what's next. Keep in mind, each person is different, and some women may not feel low during this time, but for many, rest is essential here. This is a wonderful time to spend in silence and solitude, rooting yourself in prayer to see what God might be leading you to.

FOLLICULAR PHASE (SPRING: A TIME TO DANCE)

Praise God for the follicular phase! As mentioned before, estrogen wakes up and gets the party started around day 5. From days 6 to 13, the hypothalamus (a part of your brain) receives the wake-up call and releases the gonadotropin-releasing hormone (GnRH) in response. GnRH then signals the pituitary gland (the hormone-producing factory) to release the follicle-stimulating hormone (FSH). FSH surges to the ovaries and stimulates the growth of follicles containing immature eggs. Isn't it amazing how they all work together?

You might be thinking, "What the heck is a follicle? Immature eggs? What is going on?"

Let's dive into the anatomy of the female body for a moment. You have two ovaries, one positioned to the right of the uterus and one to the left. Connecting the ovaries to the uterus are the fallopian tubes. These tubes are the pathway that allows an egg, which is housed in the ovaries, to get to the uterus, which is where a fertilized egg implants and develops into a baby.

Inside both ovaries are follicles containing eggs. Think of a jar full of marbles, but instead of glass, the jar is more like a soft sac. Inside the sac, immature eggs (eggs not ready to be used yet) await the stimulation from FSH to grow and mature. As the hormone FSH surges, the eggs grow, and one egg takes the lead, telling the rest they don't have to grow anymore. This egg is called the dominant egg. From there, the ovaries wait for the green light to release the egg into the fallopian tubes, where it begins its journey to the uterus.

"Hype girl" estrogen is working her tail off alongside FSH to get an egg ready. She is moving and grooving, making you feel confident and capable of conquering the world. As she rises, you'll likely notice a boost in energy, confidence, and clarity. This is why you often feel your best in the days right after your period. Estrogen brings out your natural glow, fuels your workouts, sharpens creativity, and even heightens your sense of desire and connection. She's all about helping you feel strong, capable, and ready to take on the world.

Known as your "spring," a time to dance, the follicular phase is the best time to push yourself, whether that's stepping it up in a workout or stepping out in faith to join a small group. If you're anything like me and love having a full social life but become drained easily, the follicular phase is the perfect time to load up your schedule. Physiologically speaking, you're most equipped to handle a large amount of stress and commitment during this time. As your body is bursting forth with new life, use this time to ask the Lord what He wants to bring forth in you. Maybe it's starting a podcast, hosting a Bible study, or joining a serve team. Maybe He's drawing your heart to go on a mission trip or start a business. Whatever prayers you've been praying and dreams you've been dreaming, press into them here and watch what God does.

OVULATORY PHASE (SUMMER: A TIME TO EMBRACE)

Welcome to the ovulatory phase! Remember how I said you can group your cycle into two halves? The ovulatory phase is what transitions one into the other. This phase is short and sweet, lasting only a few days, but buckle up because things are about to get spicy: Estrogen is at her peak, and testosterone swoops in to make you feel like you want to make a baby! This is where the Lord blows my mind, because it's not by chance that we feel the most sensual during ovulation. Even if we don't want to or can't make babies, the design is still a beautiful thing. It's also not by chance that high levels of estrogen make us feel our sexiest and most confident. Now, I know not all of us are married, and for women practicing purity, this phase can be challenging. (I have a message for you at the end of this chapter.)

During this part of your cycle, the dominant egg is finally ready to be released. The same gland that made FSH now sends a surge of luteinizing hormone (LH) to spark the release of the dominant egg from the ovary into the fallopian tube. It's a slow journey to the uterus, but this journey is what marks your fertility window. Ovulation typically lasts twelve to twenty-four hours (around day 14), but the fertility window can last anywhere from three to five days.

If you're trying to get pregnant, now is the time to take it to the bedroom!

As the egg travels to the uterus, the endometrium (uterine lining) thickens in preparation for fertilization. If fertilization happens during the journey, the next step is for the egg to implant into the uterine lining to develop a baby. Pretty miraculous, right?

This phase as known as your "summer," a time to embrace, because it's the hottest time of the month, physically and physiologically. The "hype girl," estrogen, brings the heat! No, really. You may notice that your body temperature rises slightly, you sweat more easily, and you even crave cold, refreshing foods and drinks. Biologically, your cervical mucus becomes more fertile, your libido naturally increases, and your body is primed for connection and intimacy.

Just like in the follicular phase, your body can handle heavier loads of stress and more demanding tasks during this window. It's an ideal time to schedule important conversations, presentations, or projects that require more energy and confidence. Creativity and communication flow more freely here, making this a powerful phase for stepping into leadership, teaching a class or skill, or attending social events.

Spiritually, this can be a time to use that surge of energy and confidence to pray bold prayers and engage in intercession with courage. Think of this as a season of fruitfulness—both physically, as ovulation makes conception possible, and spiritually, as your prayers and actions can sow seeds that multiply. And of course if you're married and trying to have kids, be fruitful and multiply!

LUTEAL PHASE (FALL: A TIME TO PLANT)

Some people love the luteal phase; some people dread it. It's certainly not without its challenges, but the luteal phase often gets a bad rap. This phase makes up the second half of your menstrual cycle, lasting anywhere from ten to fourteen days. If you struggle with PMS, this is where symptoms will start to appear. While estrogen was the star of the show in the follicular and ovulatory phases, progesterone steals the spotlight in the luteal. The "hype girl" needs a break, so her sister steps in and begins pumping the brakes.

Remember that jar full of marbles? The follicle, or sac that once contained an egg, comes back in a remarkable way. After releasing the egg, the follicle transforms into the corpus luteum, a temporary but powerful hormone-producing structure. Its main job is to secrete progesterone, the "chill girl" hormone that plays a critical role in preparing and sustaining the womb for new life. Progesterone keeps the lining of the uterus nutrient-rich and hospitable, creating the perfect environment for an embryo to implant and thrive.

If implantation occurs, the embryo produces human chorionic gonadotropin (hCG). When you take a pregnancy test, it's the detection of hCG that produces a positive result.

But progesterone isn't just a pregnancy hormone—it's a key player in everyday well-being. Progesterone ensures that the uterine lining functions properly, supports hormone balance, and protects against estrogen dominance. It also plays a role in thyroid health, metabolic stability, and resilience to stress.

Think of it as the body's built-in mood stabilizer. Adequate levels of progesterone have a calming effect on the brain because it helps stimulate gamma-aminobutyric acid (GABA) receptors—the same neurotransmitters involved in reducing anxiety and promoting restful sleep. This is why progesterone is the "chill" hormone: It can ease irritability, lower stress, and even help you feel more emotionally steady in the second half of your cycle.

When levels of progesterone are too low, the opposite can occur: sore breasts, cramps, irritability, mood swings—the list goes on and on. That's because progesterone acts as a counterbalance to estrogen. Too much estrogen in the body can be linked to worsening symptoms of PMDD, PCOS, and irregular cycles.

The luteal phase is known as "fall," a time to plant. After the high energy of ovulation, your hormones naturally shift, leading you to turn inward and become more in tune with your emotions. Maybe you can attest to this. Can you tell when you've crossed into the luteal phase? Maybe you feel snappier or more impatient with things that wouldn't normally bother you. Maybe you feel like you need to leave an event early because your social battery drains faster. Or maybe sitting down to read the Bible feels more difficult than usual. This season may feel heavy at times, but it's also deeply purposeful. It's a reminder to honor your boundaries, plant seeds in prayer, and trust that God is still at work even in the quieter moments.

This is a great time to take inventory of your life. What's going well? What isn't? What needs to change or be removed from your life? Is there anything new you want to try? When you're partnered with the Holy Spirit, this is a beautiful time for reflection and sanctification. You may even feel a prompting from God to revisit past hurts so you can be honest about any lingering resentment or forgiveness you've withheld. Whatever it is for you, don't shy away from the uncomfortable—that's where God does amazing things. Just like in fall when seeds are planted in faith for a future harvest, this is a time to slow down, sow intentionally into your spiritual and emotional health, and trust that God is at work beneath the surface, drawing your roots deep into fertile soil.

God's design for your body is unbelievable, huh? I'm still speechless at how He works everything together. Every organ, every hormone, every fiber of our body works to create a marvelous symphony that gives glory to our Father. Just as Ecclesiastes 3 declares that there's a season for everything, our cycles reveal the space God holds for our ups and downs, our rhythms of work and rest, and our moments of breaking down so that new growth can take root.

In the chapters ahead, we'll explore hormone imbalances in depth, discover how to care for our bodies with intention in each phase, and learn to live in harmony with our hormones.

THE CROSSROADS OF DESIRE AND DISCIPLINE

Walking in purity is hard to do in a world with endless access to pornographic content and in a culture that glorifies sex. In a hypersexualized world, it's difficult to keep our eyes locked on the Word of God, which clearly tells us to live a countercultural life. And when you're ovulating, it's even harder.

Your sex drive is at its highest thanks to estrogen mixed with a splash of testosterone. You feel confident and bold and social. Say you're single and attending worship night at a friend's house and immediately hit it off with a cute guy. Your flesh may think, "I want to hook up with him. We could just do it and repent later; it's not that big of a deal." But the Spirit says, "Resist the temptation. Remain holy as I am holy. Lean on Me and I'll give you strength to get through it." That tension is real and something every believer will feel in one form or another. But it's especially frustrating during ovulation when your body is biologically wired for connection and intimacy. Desire is a natural feeling and nothing to be ashamed about, but you must be careful not to let *fleshly desire* drive your decisions. After all, God invented sex, but He created it with boundaries in place, not to make our lives difficult but to protect us. Within marriage, intimacy is a beautiful gift that fosters connection, unity, and even new life. It's an act of worship! Outside His design, however, what was meant for good can quickly bring brokenness, confusion, and pain. God's boundaries are an expression of His love, a way of reminding us that true freedom and joy are always found inside His will.

Before I met the Lord and my husband, I crossed boundaries and made decisions I woke up regretting. I was addicted to self-pleasure for five years. I slept with boyfriends. If I could go back in time and tell myself one thing, it would be that the short moments of pleasure are not worth the years of emotional and physical turmoil that follow. Purity isn't pretending you don't feel desire; it's about surrendering that feeling to the One who created it and asking Him to help you navigate it. God's design for sex in marriage was *always* meant to be protective. He's not trying to rob you of joy; He's preserving sexual intimacy for its rightful time and place. Yes, it will take discipline. Yes, it will take boundaries. Yes, it can be hard. But you are strong and capable because of His strength and power working in you.

As a now-married woman who rewaited for years, I have a unique perspective on purity. I'm not writing this as someone who walked in purity perfectly (I didn't), but I am writing from a place of sisterly wisdom. I don't want you to have to learn the hard way like I did. And can I tell you how proud I am of you for even taking the steps to remain pure? God is even prouder. This is a journey that *needs* to be accompanied by His grace. Too often in this walk we let guilt and shame bind us, but remember what Romans 8:1 says: "Therefore, there is now no condemnation for those who are in Christ Jesus." There may be times when you slip up—that's a part of life—so etch this verse into your heart to help keep you on the right path.

From a practical standpoint, here are some ways you can combat sexual temptation:

→ Flee. Literally get up and go somewhere else. The Bible instructs us to "flee from sexual immorality" (1 Corinthians

6:18). Physically removing yourself not only creates a barrier between you and the other person but also helps bring your mind back into focus. Go for a walk or do some jumping jacks if you need to shake off the pent-up energy.

- Recite Scripture out loud. It's hard to fall into sin when the Word is on your tongue.
- Fast. If you find that you can't overcome the temptation, fast for however long the Lord prompts (without being unhealthy and, if needed, approved by a medical professional).
- Become self-disciplined in a different area of your life. Sometimes proving to yourself that you have the strength to follow through is motivation for the bigger mountains. It could be adopting a new habit like flossing every night or waking up and reading a chapter of the Bible daily.
- Make sure you're getting enough sleep at night (seven to eight hours). When you're sleep deprived, your endocrine system is thrown for a loop and your cortisol spikes. That can lead you to make decisions you wouldn't make if you were well rested.
- Move your body. Because your hormones are at their peak, getting regular exercise helps release energy. It can aid in taming the strong feelings of lust and desire.
- Pray. Remaining steadfast in prayer keeps you focused on the King and not the thing. When you're weak, Christ's power is made perfect.
- Rely on mentors, leaders, or your community for accountability and encouragement. You were never meant to do life alone, and you need extra support from people you trust to hold you accountable and speak life into you.

I believe in you, sister. You've got this. And if you slip up, don't let the Enemy prevent you from running back to the Father. Repent and keep moving forward. I'm so excited to hear the testimonies of how God strengthened you to remain obedient to His design.

PRACTICAL APPLICATION

- → Use a journal or app to observe how your energy, emotions, and focus shift throughout the month, aligning your activities with your body's natural rhythms.
- → During your menstrual phase, embrace rest and reflection, treating it as a time for renewal and spiritual recalibration.
- → Use the follicular and ovulatory phases to tackle big projects, connect socially, and pursue new opportunities with confidence and creativity.
- → In the luteal phase, slow down, reflect, and focus on emotional and spiritual growth, trusting God's work in quieter moments.
- → Reflect on how your body mirrors creation's rhythms, deepening gratitude for God's intricate and intentional craftsmanship.

SCRIPTURE TO MEDITATE ON

- → "Therefore, there is now no condemnation for those who are in Christ Jesus." (Romans 8:1)

→ "For everything there is a season, a time for every activity under heaven. A time to be born and a time to die. A time to plant and a time to harvest. A time to kill and a time to heal. A time to tear down and a time to build up. A time to cry and a time to laugh. A time to grieve and a time to dance. A time to scatter stones and a time to gather stones. A time to embrace and a time to turn away. A time to search and a time to quit searching. A time to keep and a time to throw away. A time to tear and a time to mend. A time to be quiet and a time to speak. A time to love and a time to hate. A time for war and a time for peace." (Ecclesiastes 3:1–8 NLT)

THREE

YOU'RE NOT CRAZY, YOUR HORMONES ARE IMBALANCED

UP TO 80 PERCENT OF WOMEN SUFFER FROM A HORMONE IMBALANCE at some point in their life. Some women live with these imbalances without even knowing it, and according to Northwell Health, a whopping "70 percent are unaware of conditions like PCOS that may have manifested due to hormonal irregularities."[1] This means that most women are walking around moody, bloated, anxious, or even depressed without realizing there's a reason behind it. Alisa Vitti, founder of the Cycle Syncing Method and author of *In the FLO* and *WomanCode* reveals shocking statistics about hormonal imbalances:

- One in nine women struggle with PCOS.
- One in ten women (over eight million in the US) have endometriosis.

- Eight in ten women struggle with fibroids before age fifty.
- Eight in ten women suffer from perimenopause symptoms.[2]
- One in five couples are unable to get pregnant after one year of trying.[3]

These numbers are more than just stats—they represent women like you and me, navigating battles with pain, grief, confusion, and unanswered questions. It's overwhelming to consider how many of us are silently carrying around the weight of a hormonal imbalance without any sense of direction. As cliché as it is to hear "you're not alone" over and over, it's true. Read those numbers again. You don't have to face this in isolation when there's an army of women ready to link arms with you as you walk the path of healing.

WHAT IS A HORMONAL IMBALANCE?

Hormonal imbalances occur when there's too much or too little of one or more hormones in the blood. Because hormones regulate nearly all bodily processes—sleep, mood, metabolism, growth, fertility, and even stress response—imbalances can show up in many different ways. Symptoms might include irregular periods, weight fluctuations, hair loss or excess hair growth, fatigue, acne, infertility, hot flashes, or mood swings. Even subtle imbalances can have a profound impact on daily life. Think of the endocrine system as an orchestra and hormones as musicians. When one musician plays too fast, too slow, or out of tune, it throws off the entire symphony. Hormones are delicate, but they're amazing when working as they should. Addressing hormone imbalances often involves a holistic approach, including nutrition, stress management, movement, sleep optimization, and sometimes medical interventions or supplementation. Restoring balance is much like tuning an orchestra—when every musician (hormone) is playing in harmony, the result is a beautiful, well-functioning system that allows the body to thrive. Testing for imbalances can be done through blood, saliva, or urine, each providing different insights.

WHAT CAUSES HORMONAL IMBALANCES?

A multitude of factors can cause hormones to go off course, but here are some of the most common offenders.

Chronic Stress: Prolonged periods of stress, whether caused by work, parenting, school, chronic tardiness, grief, or other aspects of life are linked to elevated cortisol. When cortisol, the hormone that helps you manage stress, remains high for too long, your body stays in a state of survival (fight or flight). Imagine that there's an alarm system in your body that goes off every time it perceives a threat. This could be from drinking caffeine on an empty stomach or a car suddenly swerving in front of you on the road. Too much of this stress for too long puts a heavy burden on your body. This is harmful because a hormonal imbalance can suppress reproductive function. Your body won't have much energy to put into making a baby or regulating a menstrual cycle if it thinks it's in survival mode.

Lack of Sleep: Did you know that while you sleep your immune system is patrolling your insides, hauling away any junk left behind from the day? While you're dreaming, your immune system is working to keep you at your healthiest. Macrophages, the immune cells responsible for this cleanup, can't function optimally if you're sleep deprived. Lack of sleep also interferes with two hormones, leptin and ghrelin. Leptin signals the feeling of fullness, and its levels decrease when you don't get enough sleep—leading to an increase in appetite throughout the day.[4] And ghrelin, the hunger hormone, increases with sleep abnormalities, which also increases appetite. Lack of sleep also messes with the thyroid-stimulating hormone and interferes with healthy insulin production, which is linked to insulin resistance. The science is clear: You need a healthy seven to eight hours of sleep every night!

Unhealthy Diet: What we choose to put into our bodies truly matters, not only for energy but for overall well-being. Consuming a diet high in processed foods, refined sugars, and unhealthy fats can contribute to imbalanced blood sugar levels and inflammation, both of which can elevate cortisol production. Your gut health also plays a huge role here. The gut and hormones are closely connected—when one struggles, the other often does too. If your gut microbiome (the community of good bacteria living in your digestive tract) is out of balance, that can affect your mood, energy, cycles, and overall hormone health.

Lack of Exercise: When it comes to movement, balance is everything—not too much, but not too little. Movement helps your body fight insulin resistance, reduces stress, helps regulate your cycle, and boosts hormones like serotonin, growth hormone, and testosterone. Yet in today's world, it's easier than ever to slip into a sedentary lifestyle. With an increase in remote work, endless digital convenience, and the ability to meet most of our needs with the swipe of a finger, many of us simply aren't moving enough. According to the World Health Organization, one in three adults do not meet the recommended physical activity levels and have a 30 to 50 percent higher chance of developing cancer, heart disease, and more.[5]

Products: Most of us wouldn't think twice before spraying perfume, putting on makeup, or choosing a cute new outfit, but everything you consume or put on your body has an effect on your hormones. Unfortunately, many cleaning products, beauty and skincare products, perfumes, and shower items are made with toxic, harmful, endocrine-disrupting chemicals—parabens and phthalates. Parabens are synthetic preservatives added to products to prevent mold growth, but they also act like estrogen in the body, disrupting natural hormone balance. Similarly, phthalates—often hidden under the label "fragrance"—mimic estrogen and interfere with the endocrine system. Both chemicals send confusing signals to your hormones because of their estrogen-like structure.

Plastics: Reducing your use of plastic is not all about saving the turtles; humans need saving too! The most toxic component of plastic is bisphenol A (BPA), which is a significant endocrine disruptor. It's found in water bottles, plastic containers, metal canned goods, and anything packaged in plastic. It's especially harmful for women trying to conceive or who are pregnant, as BPA can penetrate the placenta and enter the baby's system, increasing their risk of illness. Plastics like polyester, the main fabric in some of our clothing, are harmful. Think about this: You're doing a workout in your polyester pants and are generating a lot of sweat and heat in your privates. That heat is essentially warming up the plastic, which can be absorbed through the skin on the most intimate parts of your body. The materials in our clothing are often overlooked and deserve more attention as a link to hormonal imbalances.

Birth Control: Birth control can be a direct offender when it comes to hormone health. The oral combination pill shuts down the communication between your brain and ovaries, suppressing vital hormone production. And while different forms of birth control use different synthetic hormones, it's important to first understand how your own hormones function. See the end of this chapter for a full breakdown of how birth control works as well as pros and cons.

Alcohol: The liver plays an important role in processing excess estrogen, and alcohol can increase levels of estrogen and other hormones in the body.[6] It can also deplete your body of magnesium, a mineral that helps to manage cramps and low progesterone–related symptoms.[7] According to a study done by the National Institutes of Health, one drink a day can increase the chance of having PMS symptoms by up to 45 percent, rising to 79 percent for those who drink heavily.[8] The liver works diligently day and night, filtering out and breaking down countless substances that enter our bodies—from environmental toxins to the natural byproducts of digestion. It's one of the most resilient and forgiving organs we have, yet it is not invincible. When alcohol is added to the mix, it becomes one more burden for the liver to process, often at the expense of its other vital functions. Over time, this can lead to fatigue, sluggishness, and even more significant health concerns.

Genetics and Epigenetics: Thanks to new research in epigenetics—the study of how behaviors and environment can influence the way our genes work, without changing the DNA sequence itself—we now know that babies in utero can inherit patterns of stress, resilience, and even trauma.[9] While genetic mutations can play a role in hormonal imbalances, it's encouraging to know that our choices matter. Genetics may write the script, but it's our lifestyle—the way we nourish our bodies, manage stress, and care for our health—that has far more power over how the story unfolds.

Underlying Issues from Other Illnesses: Certain cancers and autoimmune diseases can lead to hormonal imbalances, so it's crucial to work with your healthcare provider to address the root issue first.

HOW DO I KNOW IF I HAVE A HORMONAL IMBALANCE?

With so many factors influencing your hormones, you may wonder, "How can I know if something is off?" The signs and symptoms will vary depending on which hormones are out of balance, but some general signs include the following:

- Unexplained weight gain or loss
- Irregular or missing periods
- Fatigue or low energy
- Mood swings, anxiety, or depression
- PMS that affects daily life
- Insomnia
- Changes in appetite or digestion
- Brain fog or trouble concentrating
- Frequent headaches
- Painful ovulation or periods
- Balding or thinning hair

If you identify with any of these symptoms, I encourage you to seek guidance from a trusted professional. It's important to honor the signals your body is sending and give yourself permission to pursue healing. In the next pages, we'll look at specific imbalances and learn ways to manage symptoms. As you read, keep a heart posture of grace and balance. The goal isn't to cut out every "bad" thing and eliminate foods you love, but rather to add more nourishing foods and life-giving practices that support your hormones so that over time you can enjoy treats in moderation without guilt or fear. Balance can look like swapping soda for sparkling water during the week but still sharing dessert with friends on the weekends. It can also look like eating gluten-free bread (if it helps you) during the week but still savoring delicious deep-dish pizza with your family on the weekends.

Healing isn't an all-or-nothing journey; it's a rhythm of wise choices that makes room for both health and joy. With that in mind, let's dive into the five most common hormonal imbalances so you can better understand what might be going on in your body.

FIVE OF THE MOST COMMON HORMONAL IMBALANCES

LOW ESTROGEN

Possible Causes

- High stress, resulting in high cortisol levels
- Disordered eating
- Nutrient deficiencies due to poor dietary practices or poor absorption
- Birth control
- Natural aging process
- Overexercising, especially in conjunction with calorie restriction

Possible Symptoms

- Irregular periods
- Amenorrhea (missing period)
- Low sex drive
- Vaginal dryness
- Painful sex
- Hot flashes or night sweats

- Joint pain
- Dry skin and eyes
- Depression
- Melasma (skin condition)
- Poor cognitive function, most notably poor memory
- Bright pink period blood

The Protocol for Boosting Estrogen

To naturally support estrogen production, aim to eat foods rich in phytoestrogens—plant compounds that can gently mimic estrogen's effects in the body. Good options include edamame, tempeh, natural soy (rather than processed forms), miso, flaxseeds, chickpeas, lentils, almonds, walnuts, cruciferous vegetables, and garlic. These foods contain isoflavones, which research has shown may help ease menopausal symptoms like hot flashes while also supporting bone and heart health.[10] You'll also want to ensure you're getting enough vitamins and minerals, specifically the following:

- Vitamin B, which helps your body create and use estrogen
- Vitamin D, which plays a role in estrogen synthesis
- Vitamin E, which research shows may help reduce hot flashes and insomnia[11]

Regular, moderate exercise can help regulate hormone levels and improve insulin sensitivity, which affect estrogen balance. Restorative sleep, proper stress management, and your gut health are equally important since your microbiome helps regulate the estrobolome, the part of your gut that metabolizes estrogen. As you make choices to support estrogen production, invite Jesus into the process. Pray over your meals, your movements, and your quiet times, and ask Him to guide you toward balance.

HIGH ESTROGEN

High estrogen (sometimes called estrogen dominance) is one of the most common hormonal imbalances I see in my peers and clients, and it's one I also struggle with. Estrogen dominance doesn't always mean estrogen is sky-high; it means the ratio of estrogen to progesterone is out of balance in the luteal phase, either because estrogen is elevated, progesterone is too low, or both. In functional medicine spaces, an optimal progesterone-to-estradiol ratio (Pg:E2) is generally considered to fall between 100:1 and 500:1.[12] This isn't a diagnostic tool but a way to understand how progesterone and estrogen work together—and how symptoms often correlate with this ratio.

Possible Causes

- Prolonged stress, causing high cortisol, which lowers progesterone output and blocks progesterone receptors
- Excessive alcohol consumption
- Excessive amounts of visceral fat—the fat surrounding your organs
- Low-functioning liver

- High toxin load from foods and everyday products (xenoestrogens)
- Birth control

Possible Symptoms

- Weight gain, especially in the hips and thighs
- Menstrual migraines
- Irregular periods
- Moodiness and frequent meltdowns
- Depression or weepiness
- Midcycle pain
- Brain fog
- Heavy bleeding
- Breast tenderness or cysts
- PMS or PMDD
- Fibroids
- Endometriosis
- Being overweight or obese
- Purple or blue period blood with a lot of clots

The Protocol for Lowering Estrogen

The liver plays a huge role in estrogen detoxification, and when this elimination pathway gets jammed, that can leave excess estrogen circulating in your body. Foods like cruciferous veggies can aid in flushing out excess estrogen.[13] Fiber-rich foods can do the same through the digestive tract. Flaxseeds are a great choice as they can help balance estrogen by supporting estrogen metabolism. At the same time, you may want to consider reducing or eliminating things like alcohol, caffeine, processed foods, and refined sugars, since these can place extra stress on your system.

Working to balance blood sugar is a game changer for managing excess estrogen. Blood sugar affects many vital processes in your body, including estrogen processing. An overload of estrogen can disrupt blood sugar balance, potentially leading to insulin resistance. And insulin resistance increases the risk of developing type 2 diabetes and other metabolic conditions.

Exercise is also important for blood sugar balance and optimal estrogen detox. If you struggle with balancing your blood sugar, going for a ten-minute walk after each meal can help your body improve insulin resistance and encourage hormone balance.

Also be on the lookout for sneaky parabens, phthalates, and BPAs in your everyday products: candles, perfumes, clothing, skincare products, makeup, deodorant, laundry detergent, haircare products, food storage, and cookware. Little by little, swapping to hormone-friendly products can help you walk in hormonal harmony. Here are some starting points:

- → Use glass or stainless steel instead of plastics for food storage and water bottles.
- → Swap fragrance-based products for fragrance-free or essential oil–based ones.
- → Use natural cleaning solutions for household products and laundry instead of harsh chemicals like ammonia.

- Opt for stainless steel cookware and bakeware instead of nonstick pans that include Teflon and other forever chemicals.
- Purchase aluminum-free deodorant and perfumes free of phthalates.
- Use a water filtration system to remove any heavy metals.
- Buy USDA Organic and non-GMO products whenever possible.
- Switch out polyester undergarments for 100 percent cotton ones.

Considering all these lifestyle swaps can feel overwhelming, but start small and take it one step at a time. Do your sustainable best. The key to lasting change is to make achievable, measurable goals that don't stress you out but rather motivate you to keep going. The last thing you need is more pressure and stress, which will have the opposite effect of what you're hoping to accomplish.

LOW PROGESTERONE

It's common to have a combination of high estrogen and low progesterone. Sometimes progesterone is considered "low" because it's out of proportion to estrogen, and other times it's genuinely low all on its own—both scenarios create symptoms of imbalance.

Possible Causes

- Long-term stress
- High cortisol

- Xenoestrogens
- Birth control
- Natural aging process
- Nutritional deficiencies
- Lack of sleep
- Excessive alcohol consumption
- Pregnancy complications

Possible Symptoms

- Difficulty getting or staying pregnant
- Breakthrough bleeding during the second half of the menstrual cycle
- PMS or PMDD
- Menstrual migraines
- Lack of ovulation
- A heavier flow during menstruation
- Irregular cycles and short cycles
- Bloating in the abdomen
- Swollen or painful breasts
- Brown spotting or brown period blood
- Anxiety and irritability
- Trouble sleeping
- Depression or mood swings

The Protocol for Boosting Progesterone

Progesterone, as we learned, is the "calming hormone" because of its ability to balance mood, reduce anxiety, and prepare the body for healthy cycles and pregnancy. To support its production, prioritize whole, nutrient-dense foods that stabilize blood sugar, lower inflammation, support ovulation, and help eliminate excess estrogen. Think healthy fats like avocado, wild-caught salmon, olive oil, and chia seeds to help lower inflammation. Add magnesium-rich foods, including dark, leafy greens (spinach, kale, mixed greens), to support blood sugar balance. For ovulation support, try pumpkin seeds, oysters, lentils, and grass-fed beef. To support hormone metabolism, try vitamin B6–rich foods such as chicken, turkey, bananas, and sweet potatoes. And finally, incorporate cruciferous veggies to help eliminate excess estrogen. If you follow a specific diet such as vegetarian or no seafood, you may not be getting some of these vitamins and nutrients. If that's the case, talk to your medical professional about possibly adding supplements.

Remember, the empty follicle that released the egg (called the corpus luteum) is what produces progesterone. That means supporting healthy ovulation is key to supporting healthy progesterone levels. For some women, nutrition and lifestyle shifts can make a big difference; for others, additional support may be needed. You may want to explore bioidentical hormone replacement therapy or other interventions with your medical provider. There isn't a one-size-fits-all approach—the best path is the one that helps your body thrive and brings your hormones back into balance.

THE PREGNENOLONE STEAL

Did you know your body uses the same raw materials to make both cortisol and progesterone? If you're constantly stressed, your body may prioritize cortisol production. When cortisol goes high, progesterone gets shy. This is called the pregnenolone steal. Pregnenolone is a master hormone made from cholesterol in the adrenal glands. It's a hormone building block because it gets converted into many other hormones, including progesterone, dehydroepiandrosterone (DHEA), testosterone, estrogen, and cortisol. When under chronic stress, your body prioritizes survival. This means that the adrenal glands crank out more cortisol to keep up with the constant demand and, in doing so, "steal" pregnenolone and diverts it to cortisol production, leaving less of it available for progesterone. This process may seem overwhelming, but it's beautiful that God created our bodies to keep us safe and protect us from harm. Even in survival mode, your body does all it can to equip you to tackle the stressor. That's an incredible gift from the Lord.

Although stress is sometimes out of your control, you can still bring Jesus into your daily routines and pray for peace. Here are some ideas:

- Meditate on Scripture and recite it throughout the day. A great verse to start with is 2 Timothy 1:7 (NKJV): "For God has not given us a spirit of fear, but of power and of love and of a sound mind."
- Hold every thought captive and reframe your negative thought or fear to align with God's truth. Example: "I can't

stop worrying about the results of my scan." Reframe: "I can do all things because God is with me and gives me strength. With Him I don't need to be afraid, no matter what the results say."

- → Take ten minutes out of your day to go for a prayer walk.
- → Share your burdens with a friend or mentor. According to a study from the University of Michigan, feeling emotionally close to a friend increases levels of progesterone.[14] This makes Galatians 6:2 even more divine—sharing each other's burdens fulfills the law of Christ.

Diving Deeper: PMDD

Premenstrual dysphoric disorder (PMDD) is a severe hormone sensitivity disorder affecting up to 10 percent of menstruating women. It's not just "bad PMS"; it's an exhausting condition that causes women to experience severe mood swings, anger, irritability, anxiety, depression, or feelings of hopelessness in the luteal phase. Fatigue, insomnia, lack of concentration, and physical symptoms like bloating, cramps, and breast tenderness also can accompany PMDD. This condition can affect relationships, jobs, motivation, social life, self-image, and even stress management. Women with PMDD (myself included) are often told that it's all in their mind—they're just "crazy"—and that having intense mental struggles in the luteal phase is normal. But it's definitely not normal.

While the root cause of PMDD is not fully known, here's what we do know: PMDD seems to be linked to the drop in estrogen and rise in progesterone during the second half of the menstrual cycle—the luteal phase. It's not clinically proven to be caused by low progesterone; in fact, a lot of women have normal progesterone levels in the luteal phase. Rather, it's the way the brain responds to the shift in hormones. These hormonal changes can cause an imbalance in neurotransmitters like serotonin, which plays a key role in mood regulation.[15] Fluctuations in estrogen and progesterone throughout the menstrual cycle directly influence serotonin activity, which is why many women experience heightened depression, anxiety, or irritability in the luteal phase. But serotonin is only part of the picture. Research shows that women with PMDD often react differently to the brain's calming system because of changes in a progesterone-derived neurosteroid called allopregnanolone.[16] Normally, allopregnanolone helps quiet the mind and ease stress, but in PMDD, the hormonal shifts can make the brain overact instead of relax. This means the very hormone that should bring calm can trigger intense emotional and physical symptoms instead. This unique interaction helps explain why PMDD symptoms can feel so overwhelming and intense compared with those of PMS.

Chronic stress, poor diet, lack of exercise, and inadequate sleep can further strain these systems, intensifying symptoms. Additionally, research shows that a history of trauma such as childhood abuse is connected to an increased vulnerability to developing PMDD. This is due to the altered stress response circuits in the brain, which make you more sensitive to these hormonal shifts.[17]

In my own life, I've noticed that increasing protein and healthy fats while reducing carbohydrates helps with not only minimizing blood sugar spikes but also regulating my mood. Nutrition and lifestyle changes can help minimize symptoms, but managing stress is often the most important thing for a woman with PMDD. This means it may be wise to lower intake of stressors like caffeine and alcohol, knowing they can increase anxiety and sleep issues, which you may already experience with this disorder. And to prevent spikes in cortisol, consider switching your workouts to low-impact movements like Pilates, walking, barre, and light strength training.

If you have PMDD, consider talking to your healthcare provider, and know you're not alone. I have struggled with PMDD since adolescence, and it's one of the reasons you're holding this book today. I spent decades believing there was something wrong with me, but after countless hours researching and trying holistic remedies to decrease my symptoms, along with talking to my OB/GYN about other alternatives, I can tell you with confidence that you are not doomed with this disorder. Etch Isaiah 40:4 on your heart:

> Every valley shall be raised up,
>   every mountain and hill made low;
> the rough ground shall become level,
>   the rugged places a plain.

God can bring balance where things feel off-kilter and calm where your body feels chaotic. Nothing about your hormones or healing journey is too difficult or too heavy for Him to redeem.

EXCESS ANDROGENS

Possible Causes

- High insulin levels, which cause the ovaries to produce more testosterone
- Hormonal birth control with synthetic progestins
- Polycystic ovary syndrome (PCOS)
- High cortisol from chronic stress
- Excess body fat, which can cause excess estrogen, which can affect the production and use of androgens in women
- Congenital adrenal hyperplasia

Possible Symptoms

- Unstable blood sugar, known as hypo- or hyperglycemia
- Infrequent ovulation
- Menstrual cycles longer than thirty-five days
- Ovarian cysts
- Midcycle pain
- Acne or oily skin
- Weight gain
- Hair growth on the face or other unwanted areas
- Hair loss on the head

Diving Deeper: PCOS

Since PCOS is the most common condition linked to excess androgens, let's take a closer look at what it is and explore practical ways to help ease its symptoms. Polycystic ovary syndrome (PCOS) is both a hormonal imbalance and a metabolic disorder caused by excess androgens that can cause weight gain, hair growth in unwanted areas, infertility, acne, and ovarian cysts. It affects an estimated 13 percent of reproductive-aged women worldwide, and up to 70 percent of those women aren't getting diagnosed and thus are not receiving the treatment they need.[18] It can take women three to five years to receive a diagnosis, a devastating reality that needs to change. Left untreated, PCOS can lead to infertility, weight gain, cardiovascular disease, diabetes, depression, and a whole host of other hormone-related issues. Because of a lack of research, we don't know what causes it, but it's suggested that it develops from a combination of genetic, hormonal, and metabolic factors. These often occur alongside irregular periods (anovulation). For example, 70 percent or more of women with PCOS have insulin resistance, in which the ovaries react to the excess insulin by stimulating theca cells, which in turn produce higher amounts of testosterone.[19] This creates a vicious cycle—elevated testosterone levels can worsen insulin resistance, and worsening insulin resistance can drive testosterone even higher.

Learning about PCOS can feel overwhelming, and to make matters more confusing, there's a lot of misinformation floating around online and in social circles. These myths not only cause unnecessary fear but also prevent women from understanding the truth about their bodies. Jolene Brighten, a board certified naturopathic endocrinologist and leading expert in PCOS, shares a few myths about PCOS:

→ You must have cysts on your ovaries to be diagnosed.

- Weight gain causes PCOS. (Rather, it's a symptom.)[20]
- Birth control is the only treatment option.
- Everyone with PCOS is overweight.[21]

You can see that PCOS isn't as black-and-white as it seems. If you've ever been unfairly stereotyped, my heart breaks for you. Maybe someone told you, "You just need to lose weight," or dismissed your pain by saying, "That's just part of being a woman." Maybe you've been misunderstood at the doctor's office, brushed off by friends or family, or even judged for symptoms outside of your control. That's an isolating and heavy feeling, and I'm so sorry if this has been your experience.

But here's the good news: PCOS does have clear diagnostic criteria, which can bring both answers and relief. According to the Rotterdam criteria, diagnosing PCOS requires the presence of two of these three symptoms:

- Ovulatory dysfunction (missing periods or irregular periods more than forty-five days in length)
- Excess androgens
- Polycystic ovaries or elevated anti-Mullerian hormone levels[22]

The Protocol for PCOS

If you've been diagnosed with or suspect you have PCOS, your nutritional focus should be getting protein, plants, and healthy fat in every single meal. Protein is essential for those with PCOS, even more so for those over thirty-five because as you age, your muscle mass decreases, putting you at higher risk of cardiometabolic disease. For those with PCOS, muscle is one of the most important metabolic organs to use as leverage. Aim for 1 to 1.2 grams of protein per kilogram of body weight to maintain muscle mass, optimize blood sugar, and experience fullness after meals. You should also eat colorful vegetables for their phytonutrients, in addition to fiber (aim for 25 grams daily). Fiber is important not only because it makes you feel full longer but also because it slows the rate at which glucose is absorbed, leading to more balanced blood sugar levels. Fiber also helps your gut, which is crucial for lowering the amount of visceral fat around the organs. Some examples of fiber are brown rice, lentils, sweet potato, and oatmeal. But be mindful that for some, fiber can cause digestion issues, so you should always consult with your doctor to find the right foods for you.

Healthy fats are equally important because some fiber can spike blood sugar, but paired with fat and protein in healthy amounts, it won't. Healthy fats include avocado, chia seeds, coconut oil, and fatty fish. If you can visualize a plate, half the plate should be protein, and the other half should be divided into half again for plants and carbohydrates. One to two tablespoons of healthy fat should be added to the plate as well.

Weight is a sensitive topic. Even more so for women with this condition, as it can feel impossible to lose weight. You're doing everything "right," yet nothing is working. And then there are women who aren't overweight but have hair loss, gut issues, and depression. They've tried every hair growth serum on the market and spent years on antidepressants all to feel worse than before. PCOS exists on a spectrum, and no matter where you fall on it, managing symptoms can feel hopeless. Take my suggestions with a grain of grace—you know your body better than I do—but maybe there's something here you can try.

Try getting more movement throughout the day: thirty minutes daily in ten-minute increments. Spreading it throughout your day can be less overwhelming and more effective for improving insulin resistance. Strength training is also great for those with PCOS. Muscle is one of the most insulin-sensitive tissues in the body, meaning the more muscle you have, the more effectively your body can use insulin. Pilates, low-impact movements, and body-weight exercises are fabulous and PCOS-friendly. Less is more when it comes to PCOS.

The last thing I'll mention about PCOS is birth control since it may be the first thing doctors advise you start. While it can be useful for managing some symptoms like acne, it's important to know what birth control does and doesn't do.

Birth control, especially the oral combination pill, does not restore or regulate your menstrual cycle. It shuts down the communication between your ovaries and brain, thus suppressing FSH and LH production. Without these two hormones, ovulation does not occur. This is not ideal if you're already struggling with irregular periods and infrequent ovulation, as it further suppresses this process. The bleed you do get is a withdrawal bleed, which can be powerful and necessary for some cases of PCOS. To get to progesterone, you need to pass through ovulation since progesterone is produced by the corpus luteum. Your body makes progesterone only after you ovulate. In PCOS, ovulation can be rare, so progesterone can stay low while estrogen stays relatively higher. Too much estrogen without enough progesterone can make the uterine lining keep growing, which over time can lead to endometrial hyperplasia and raise the risk of endometrial cancer. In these cases, the pill can help by stopping the lining from getting too thick and lowering that risk.

The pill can also reduce androgens (like testosterone) from the ovaries and increase a protein (sex hormone–binding globulin) that ties up extra testosterone—often improving hormonal acne.

Birth control has many pros and cons. What's important to understand is that your PCOS symptoms will likely come back when you stop hormonal birth control, and sometimes worse than before. While birth control can be a helpful tool in some cases, it's also important to note that it doesn't address the other issues PCOS is linked to, like cardiovascular disease, metabolic dysfunction, and mental health disorders. As always, consult with a medical professional to determine what is right for you. And for more detail, see page 63.

LOW ANDROGENS

Possible Causes

- → Dysfunction in the adrenal glands or the ovaries
- → Ovarian removal, low ovarian function, or ovarian failure
- → Birth control
- → Overexercising or undereating
- → Chronic stress

- Pituitary or thyroid issues
- Addison's disease
- Hypopituitarism (pituitary gland dysfunction)

Possible Symptoms

- Low libido
- Painful intercourse
- Low self-confidence
- Vaginal dryness
- Diminished muscle mass
- Decreased motivation
- Fatigue
- Irregular periods
- Thinning hair
- Depression
- Anxiety

The Protocol for Boosting Androgens

To boost androgens, focus on managing stress, getting adequate sleep, reducing caffeine intake, eating enough nutrient-dense foods, and doing strength training, which can help increase natural testosterone levels. Prioritizing protein and healthy fats such as salmon, grass-fed meats, olive oil, avocado, and nuts provides the building blocks your body needs for hormone production. Minerals like magnesium and zinc, found in foods such as oysters, pumpkin seeds, and leafy greens, are especially important for DHEA and testosterone synthesis. For some women, a doctor may recommend low-dose DHEA supplementation, especially in cases of adrenal insufficiency or fertility challenges. Supplementation, when tailored to your unique needs and overseen by a professional, can be a bridge toward restored energy, mood, and vitality.

If you suspect you have low androgens, getting a blood test can help determine what is out of balance. Ask your doctor or functional practitioner to test your key androgen markers:

- Total and free testosterone
- DHEA-S
- Androstenedione
- Sex hormone–binding globulin (SHBG)

It's also helpful to check the following to understand your overall hormonal picture:

- FSH and LH
- Cortisol
- Estradiol
- Progesterone

Having low androgens can affect more than just your physical health—it can also impact the way you see yourself. When androgens drop, confidence, motivation, and self-esteem can drop with them. But Isaiah 61, verses 1 and 3 reminds us that God exchanges our deepest places of pain and heaviness for His beauty, joy, and praise:

> The Lord has anointed me to . . .
> provide for those who grieve in Zion—

to bestow on them a crown of beauty
  instead of ashes,
the oil of joy
  instead of mourning,
and a garment of praise.

That's exactly what Jesus does for us: He removes our heaviness and clothes us with a garment of praise. He is a good Father, ready to remind us that joy springs forth when we look to Him. Through it all, remember that God designed you intentionally. Your hormones are not broken beyond repair, and a lab result or diagnosis does not define your worth. Inviting the Lord into this healing journey is transformative. Pray for wisdom, clarity, and motivation, and trust that with patience, consistency, and faith, you can find balance in your body once again.

Whatever hormonal imbalance you may struggle with, healing is possible and joy is your portion. If God is for you, who (or what) can be against you! There's no diagnosis too big and no symptom too small for Him. Your diagnosis is not a death sentence, it's not your identity, and it doesn't have to stop you from living your life. With Jesus, anything is possible.

HOW BIRTH CONTROL WORKS

We can't continue the topic of hormonal imbalances without talking about birth control in more detail. Let me set the record straight: I am not anti–birth control, but I am all for education about birth control. A CDC study from 2015 to 2017 found that 65 percent of women ages fifteen to forty-nine used birth control. Among women ages fifteen to twenty-nine, oral contraceptives, a.k.a. the pill, were most common.[23] More than half of women in their reproductive years have taken birth control, but I bet that the majority of them were never properly informed about how it works or the potential side effects. And that's not their fault. Unfortunately, it's given out like candy in most OB/GYN offices and is often used as a bandage to cover deeper issues.

Here's how hormonal birth control works. (Keep in mind, each contraceptive method works slightly differently depending on which hormones it has, but right now I'm talking about the oral combination pill.) The pill is made of synthetic (man-made) estrogen and progesterone, which block the signal in the brain that triggers the production of follicle-stimulating hormone (FSH) and luteinizing hormone (LH). Normally, the hypothalamus acts as the messenger between the ovaries and brain. When you're in the follicular phase—the phase where your body is stimulating the growth of an egg—the hypothalamus receives the signal and releases gonadotropin-releasing hormone (GnRH), which in turn alerts the pituitary gland to make FSH and LH. Since birth control cuts the hypothalamic communication cord, there is no signal to produce these hormones. Without these hormones being produced, ovulation no longer occurs. The pill also thickens the cervical mucus, making it difficult for sperm to pass through, and thins the lining of the uterus to make implantation of a fertilized egg less probable. And again, the bleed you get while taking the pill isn't your normal period. It's called a withdrawal bleed—the result of taking a week's worth of placebo pills—and sadly, it's been falsely communicated to women that because they're bleeding monthly, their cycle is regulated.

Birth control is a powerful drug and needs to be approached with healthy caution. Many women have reported that it has taken them four to six months to regain a normal menstrual cycle after stopping birth control.[24] In my own life, after the removal of a hormonal IUD after ten years, it took my body many months to sort itself out. The journey to regaining a healthy cycle further opened my eyes to the impact birth control has on our delicate bodies.

Hormonal birth control has also been scientifically proven to deplete your body of essential vitamins and minerals, including folic acid, vitamins B2, B6, B12, C, and E, and the minerals magnesium, selenium, and zinc.[25] So if you are on the pill, it may be wise to investigate supplementing these key nutrients.

Depression, weight gain, anxiety, sleep disruption, changes in sex drive, lack of motivation to do daily tasks, a sense of not feeling like yourself anymore—these are just a few of the complaints I've heard from women online and in my own life who are currently on or had once been on birth control. A study of Danish women ages fifteen to thirty-four found that progesterone-only contraceptives—including the IUD—were associated with higher risk of depression, with the strongest effects seen in teens.[26] Though the overall number was small, it's real. And it breaks my heart to see young girls suffering from mood disorders who perhaps weren't properly informed about the risks of birth control.

Like I said, I'm not anti–birth control. In fact, going on the IUD when I was in the thick of my bleeding disorder as a teenager may have saved my life. When used properly, it can be an incredible tool for healing and relieving pain. I know of women who struggle with crippling ovarian cyst pain who need to be on birth control to function normally in society. And I know women who deal with intense hormonal acne and only found relief using the pill. My argument is that people should be fully educated about the risks of birth control, and it should be used *alongside* other methods of treatment. Where we can run into trouble is in its long-term use or when it is used to cover up underlying issues without addressing them. My OB/GYN, Dr. Lundberg, explained it to me this way: If you have irregular periods before going on birth control, you will likely struggle with irregular periods when you go off it (if you haven't utilized other methods of healing). You simply delay addressing the issue.

Let's review a scenario together. Emily has struggled with irregular periods since her first bleed at age fourteen. She would spot here and there, would get a heavy period, and then wouldn't get one at all for four months. She assumed going on birth control would regulate her cycle. Emily has now been on the pill for twenty years, has recently gotten married, and has decided she wants to start a family. To her surprise, she's having a hard time getting pregnant even though she was "regular" on the pill. Her initial issue of irregular periods has returned, and she feels defeated because nobody told her that birth control didn't fix her root issue. Emily is now in her mid-thirties and feels like she's in a race against the clock to get a healthy cycle to boost her fertility.

I don't want this to be you. But if it is, know that your story is more common than you think. I pray in Jesus's name for healing over your womb and that God blesses you in the way He answers your prayers. But the lack of education in women's health must change. And it begins with you and me using our knowledge and Spirit-led wisdom to make informed decisions about our health. Whether that means going on birth control temporarily to relieve pain, or going off it to focus on restoring your cycle, you are on your own unique journey and timeline. What matters most is that you're prayerfully seeking God's wisdom and choosing the path that best supports your health and wholeness.

WHAT'S CONSIDERED "NORMAL"?

Cycle Length: Your cycle should fall anywhere between twenty-one and thirty-five days. Anywhere in that range is fine as long as it's consistent from month to month.

Blood Color: Your bleed should be a deep red color, like cranberry juice, from start to finish. If your blood is light pink, you may have low estrogen. If it's brown, that may signal low progesterone, and if it's deep purple or blue with clots, that may signal high estrogen.

Bleed Length: You should be bleeding anywhere from three to seven days.

Flow Heaviness: Ideally, you should have a strong flow with no clots. But you shouldn't need to change your menstrual products every hour, nor should you be bleeding through products or clothes.

Physical Symptoms: It's normal and healthy to feel some sensations in your uterus but not to the point where you're racing to the medicine cabinet for pain relievers.

If you've been feeling like a stranger in your own body, snapping at people you love, crying over things you can't put language to, feeling exhausted by noon, hating what you see in the mirror, it may not be you—it may be your hormones. After what you've learned in this chapter, I hope you feel relieved and empowered, realizing there's a reason behind the chaos. You're not crazy. With knowledge comes clarity, and with clarity, hope. My prayer is that we become a generation that is well educated, properly informed, and Holy Spirit led when it comes to making decisions for our health. Proverbs 16:16 says, "How much better to get wisdom than gold, to get insight rather than silver!" May we be women who pursue wisdom with boldness and learn to treat our bodies with the reverence and care they deserve.

PRACTICAL APPLICATION

→ Determine which hormonal imbalance you may be experiencing, and try incorporating one tip from the protocol.

→ Track your symptoms week by week in a journal to get a better picture of what's going on.

→ Journal about your emotions, fears, disappointments, and goals.

SCRIPTURE TO MEDITATE ON

→ "Every valley shall be raised up, every mountain and hill made low; the rough ground shall become level, the rugged places a plain." (Isaiah 40:4)

- "How much better to get wisdom than gold, to get insight rather than silver!" (Proverbs 16:16)
- "The Lord has anointed me to . . . provide for those who grieve in Zion—to bestow on them a crown of beauty instead of ashes, the oil of joy instead of mourning, and a garment of praise." (Isaiah 61:1, 3)

FOUR

"IS IT SPIRITUAL WARFARE, OR AM I JUST GETTING MY PERIOD?"

I SAT ON THE EDGE OF MY BED, STARING AT THE CEILING, wondering why I had such a heavy weight on my chest. The PMS came out of nowhere—anxiety; depression; doubt about my faith, my career, my life. It was a sense of hopelessness I couldn't shake. I'd dealt with these feelings before and brushed them off as being a result of "one of those days," but this day felt different. The sense of doom was too real, the heaviness in my heart too weighty. It seemed as if an external force was deliberately oppressing me, and I couldn't ignore the nagging thought, "Is this spiritual warfare, or am I just getting my period?" As I sat there, unsure whether to start warring in prayer or to grab a heating pad, I realized that the answer might not be so simple.

The lines between the natural and the spiritual often feel blurred. God gifted me with a heightened sensitivity, meaning I am hyperaware of things happening in the spiritual realm that feel as if they're unfolding in front of me in the natural world. Though I can't see them with my physical eyes, I perceive them deep in my soul. And I often have difficulty determining whether my anxiety is from my social calendar or from a spiritual shift, leaving me caught in a whirlwind of uncertainty, unsure whether my emotions are truly mine or if the devil is throwing fiery arrows.

Can you relate to that feeling? Have you experienced emotions so intense that it feels like you're caught between two worlds, playing tug-of-war with the devil? Maybe you've never been able to put it into words, but you can feel in your gut a dark, sinking sensation of knowing there's a spiritual component at play. I'm sure some of you have been there, torn between what the devil is throwing at you and what your body is actually suffering from.

Through Scripture, prayer, and revelation, the Lord has opened my eyes to see clearly. Yes, spiritual warfare and PMS can happen simultaneously, and bless your heart, sister, if this is happening to you right now. But often our hormones play tricks on us, making our circumstances bigger, harder, and more overwhelming than they need to be. The fog of PMS can make every thought feel like an attack, but not every low moment is warfare—sometimes it's simply your body crying out for rest and care. And that's where God meets you tenderly. Sometimes we use the phrase "spiritual warfare" more casually than we realize, but it's worth pausing to acknowledge the true gravity of what that means. Spiritual warfare is intense and very real, and while our daily struggles matter, not every challenge reflects that same level of spiritual magnitude.

DEFINING PMS AND WARFARE

Before we go any further, let's define what these terms mean. Premenstrual syndrome (PMS) is a set of physical, emotional, and behavioral symptoms that occur in the luteal phase of the menstrual cycle (days before menstruation). Common examples include the following:

- → Emotional: irritability, mood swings, depression, anxiety
- → Physical: bloating, weight gain, cramps, breast tenderness, headaches
- → Behavioral: disrupted sleep, appetite changes, trouble concentrating

So then what is spiritual warfare? It's the battle between Satan and God's people that can manifest physically, mentally, spiritually, and psychologically. Ephesians 6:12 says, "Our struggle is not against flesh and blood, but against the rulers, against the authorities, against the powers of this dark world and against the spiritual forces of evil in the heavenly realms." The best news is that God has already defeated the devil and given us victory, but Satan still prowls around like a roaring lion looking for someone to devour (1 Peter 5:8). He's a sore loser! With our victory secured, it's important to understand what spiritual warfare truly looks like so we can recognize it when it comes and stand firm in the authority God has given us.

Here are some examples of what spiritual warfare is and is not.

Spiritual warfare is *not*:

- → Your boss micromanaging you after you've been late on deadlines
- → Your spouse becoming upset with you after you repeatedly engage in a behavior they've asked you to change
- → Feeling overwhelmed by stress due to poor time management and lack of boundaries
- → Becoming irritable and sluggish because you chose to stay up until 2:00 a.m.

Spiritual warfare *is*:

- → Believing God doesn't love you and that you're not enough
- → Carrying generational patterns of suffering (illnesses, addictions, etc.)
- → Praying for breakthrough in an area of your life but feeling as if something is pushing against you, fighting you
- → Being tempted to act against moral or biblical principles

Satan is after one thing and one thing only: your faith in God. He's not after your relationship, your ministry, or your calling—at least not directly. He shakes these up as a means to an end, but the end is always your belief in Jesus Christ as Lord and Savior. He knows that if he can distract and discourage you enough, you'll question whether God is good after all. This is why the battlefield is often in the mind and heart. He'll use the cracks—your insecurities, your weariness, your physical pain, your hormones—to try to plant seeds of doubt. His goal is not only to make life hard but to separate you from hope, to whisper lies so convincing that you forget the truth you already know: Jesus has already won the victory.

DISCERNING BETWEEN THE TWO

We've talked about the spiritual side of things, so now let's compare that with hormones and how they can influence our mental and physical health. Spiritual warfare is spiritual in nature: It is caused by external spiritual forces or internal struggles with sin; it can happen anytime, anywhere, lasting from days to months to years; and it can be addressed through Bible reading, prayer, fasting, repentance, and deliverance. PMS is biological in nature: It is caused by hormonal fluctuations during the menstrual cycle; it occurs cyclically before menstruation, lasting from a few days to two weeks; and it can be addressed by medical or lifestyle interventions (and prayer, of course!).

SPIRITUAL VERSUS BIOLOGICAL

ASPECT	SPIRITUAL WARFARE	PMS
Nature	Spiritual (related to faith and beliefs)	Biological (hormonal and physical)
Cause	External spiritual forces or internal struggles with sin	Hormonal fluctuations during the menstrual cycle
Duration	Can happen for any length of time, triggered by life circumstances or spiritual battles	Occurs cyclically before menstruation

You may be reading this rolling your eyes, saying, "I need deliverance from the demon that is my cramps!" To that I say, I hear you. There are times when my PMDD is so bad I feel like I become a different person. Perhaps you've spent hours curled around the toilet because the pain is so severe it makes you vomit, or you've made a trip to the emergency room convinced your appendix ruptured, only for the doctor to tell you that an ovarian cyst burst. I cannot express how deeply sorry I am for the physical, emotional, and mental toll that your experience has taken on you. It's more than just discomfort; it's a deep, exhausting struggle that affects every aspect of your life. Please know I truly empathize with you—your pain is seen, your frustration is understood, and you are not carrying this burden alone.

Our hormones are mind-blowingly strong and have the power to influence our mental and physical health. But hormones are not the devil. They're not evil forces deliberately wreaking havoc on our bodies; they're delicate helpers that

God designed to make us healthy and happy. How we live can help set them up for success, and I'm here to help you do that.

The beautiful thing about both warfare and PMS is that they both show us how much we need Jesus. They're two realities that can feel scary, hopeless, and out of our control. We can let the warfare and spiritual challenges weaken our armor further, or we can use them to grow closer to God. Same with our menstrual cycle: We can see it as a burden and something to despise, or we can use it as a monthly reminder that we have to rely on God for aid. In moments of trouble, we put on the armor of God and suit ourselves up with the belt of truth, the breastplate of righteousness, the shield of faith, the helmet of salvation, and the sword of the Spirit. We combat lies with truth, counter fear with faith, and resist evil with godly actions.

Ultimately, these challenges force us to confront our vulnerabilities while providing an opportunity to lean into the grace and power of God. We can choose to embrace the battles as occasions to deepen our intimacy with Him, knowing that in every trial, He equips us with what we need to stand firm. So when the spiritual warfare feels too heavy, and when your hormones make you feel like you're losing all control, remember that you're not alone in the fight, and through Christ, you're always empowered to overcome. And know there's nothing that can separate you from God's love, no matter how intense the PMS becomes or how scary the warfare may seem. Romans 8:38–39 assures us of this: "I am convinced that neither death nor life, neither angels nor demons, neither the present nor the future, nor any powers, neither height nor depth, nor anything else in all creation, will be able to separate us from the love of God that is in Christ Jesus our Lord."

Yes, it might be spiritual warfare. But it might be a lack of progesterone. The devil loves to strike when we're most vulnerable, and hormonal fluctuations can make us a target. The more we understand our design, the better suited we are to fight back with the right weapons. So the next time you feel off, ask the Holy Spirit for help—and maybe check your cycle tracker too.

PRACTICAL APPLICATION

The next time you find yourself confused about whether you're experiencing warfare or hormones, ask yourself these questions and refer to the previous table to compare results.

- When did these thoughts, beliefs, or behaviors begin?
- Did a trigger or life event cause these thoughts, beliefs, or behaviors?
- Have these thoughts, beliefs, or behaviors occurred in the past? If so, when? Is there a pattern to when they show up?
- Where am I in my menstrual cycle?
- What symptoms am I feeling in my body?
- Are these symptoms worsening as I get closer to my period?

- Can these symptoms be alleviated through lifestyle changes like diet and exercise?
- What are the negative thoughts saying? Are they about me or about God?
- Do my symptoms feel spiritual or physical?
- What is God saying about these thoughts, beliefs, or behaviors?

SCRIPTURE TO MEDITATE ON

- "I am convinced that neither death nor life, neither angels nor demons, neither the present nor the future, nor any powers, neither height nor depth, nor anything else in all creation, will be able to separate us from the love of God that is in Christ Jesus our Lord." (Romans 8:38–39)
- "Our struggle is not against flesh and blood, but against the rulers, against the authorities, against the powers of this dark world and against the spiritual forces of evil in the heavenly realms." (Ephesians 6:12)

PART TWO

GETTING TO KNOW THE WOMAN GOD MADE

FIVE

THE PAIN, THE PIT, AND THE PROCESS OF SANCTIFICATION

"I CAN'T DO THIS ANYMORE."

That was the line I kept repeating to myself as I received phone call after phone call from different doctors.

Physician. Gynecologist. Oncologist. Physician. Gynecologist. Oncologist.

Each month, there was something new and concerning with my health. If my dentist had called next to say I had a cavity, I would've thrown my phone into the Hudson River.

I'm no stranger to suffering. It's probably the one thing I'm used to. Most of my adolescent years were spent in and out of the hospital and doctors' offices, running from expert to expert to figure out what was going on with my declining health.

When I was fifteen years old, I was diagnosed with a chronic autoimmune disorder called idiopathic thrombocytopenic purpura (ITP). Say that ten times fast! A few weeks after receiving the flu shot, I developed a gnarly virus. I was achy, feverish, sore—I felt awful. I went to the doctor, and he put me on a medication that I soon learned is a cousin of a medication I'm allergic to. A few days later, I noticed little red dots covering my ankles, knees, and chest. Concerned, my mom took me back to the doctor.

I'll never forget the look of confusion mixed with panic that my primary physician had when examining my legs. He even called in two of his peers. Panic rose in me because you don't call in your peers unless something is off, right? After their examination, they explained that the red dots were called petechiae (bleeding from broken capillaries) and that I needed a blood test immediately. They were careful not to give a diagnosis prematurely but emphasized the urgency of the situation, which didn't ease my anxiety.

When my test results came back, they noted that my platelet count (platelets are what stop you from bleeding) was 12,000. A typical platelet count range is anywhere from 150,000 to 300,000. It doesn't take a mathematician to see the deficiency there. When my mom pulled me out of my varsity basketball practice early, I knew something wasn't right because her voice broke and her eyes welled up with tears as she explained that we needed to go to the hospital right away. A few hours later the pediatric oncologist came into the room to give me my diagnosis. She explained what ITP is: an autoimmune disease where your body flips on itself and starts attacking your platelets rather than harmful viruses, causing a low platelet count. This leads to excessive bruising and bleeding, causing petechiae.

What came next was a year-and-a-half-long battle to remission. Injections, steroids, pills . . . more injections, more steroids, more pills. Daily treatments lasted seven hours each. My body rejected everything that should've worked. My numbers would climb, then crash the next day. Every time I had a blood test, I awaited a disappointed look from my doctor. I was stuck in an endless cycle of a new treatment getting my hopes up only to be let down by the results. It was a weekly reminder that I am not ultimately in control of my health and my future.

"We believe chemotherapy is the best option for Kim and has the highest chance of resolving the problem."

My dad's hands shook as he signed the paperwork stating that if anything were to happen to me during treatment (that is, if I died), the hospital wasn't liable. Four rounds of nonradioactive chemotherapy were up next. I was not prepared for the strange sensations and body aches that would ensue during treatment. My body felt things it never felt before—things no teenager, or anyone, should ever have to experience. It was terrifying.

By the grace of God, I was healed. Months came and went, and my platelet count remained stabilized. No more emergency room visits, no more outpatient treatments, no more stale hospital crackers or scratchy yellow socks. Finally, I was in remission.

I didn't have a relationship with Jesus then, but I now know He's the One who healed me.

You can imagine the toll all the treatments took on

my adolescent body. Because ITP causes excess bleeding, my periods became dangerous. I was bleeding through two heavy pads *and* my pants. I was sixteen, and it was humiliating to walk down to the school nurse's office to call my mom and ask if she'd bring me new leggings. So we decided, along with my team of doctors, that going on birth control—specifically the IUD—was a necessity. I wasn't really given a choice because of the severity of my blood disease: The risk of external bleeding was high, but the risk of internal bleeding in my brain was even worse. I had to stop playing all sports, drive only short distances, and be extra cautious everywhere I went. All my freedoms were stripped from me, and the only thing I could do about it was *nothing*.

Right as I was beginning to embrace and understand my womanhood, my period was taken away completely. The IUD was wonderful and prevented what could've been dangerous situations, but I didn't have the liberty of getting to know my body and my menstrual cycle in the way I would've liked.

In addition to that loss, nobody could have prepared me for what I'd deal with in the future. Ever since my last round of treatment in 2016, I've struggled with fighting common colds, viral infections, and allergies.

Nearly a decade later, I still deal with the ripple effects of my chronic disease. Swollen lymph nodes, strange findings on MRI and CT scans, cancer scares—these are the new burdensome obstacles I face on the regular.

I've wrestled many nights asking God why He allowed me to drink this cup of suffering. Why wasn't I given a fair shot at developing a strong, healthy body? Why must I battle PTSD and fear-based nightmares about my past? And why do I *still* have to deal with these problems? Wasn't one life-threatening disease enough?

I've cried on my knees, begging Him to heal my immune system, repair what's been broken, and give me a restored body. I've fallen into depressions so low I was convinced I couldn't go on. And I've gotten so bitter that I resented the healthy people around me.

Maybe you've felt the same way. Your struggles may be like mine, or they may be radically different. You have a unique health journey with unique forms of suffering—whether that's PCOS, endometriosis, cysts, hypothyroidism, PMDD, infertility, autoimmunity, or something else. Or you might only struggle with the (often intense) challenges of a regular cycle. Either way, you've likely experienced the frustration of shaking your fist at God, crying out, "Why me?" as you've watched others effortlessly prance through life. You can probably also relate to the physical and emotional toll that comes with the pain and the many questions it stirs within you.

There's an unspoken belief in some corners of the church and among some believers that we can't mourn or be upset with God. It's true that God is working all things for our good and that He will fight our battles for us. But those promises don't mean we have to skip right over our sadness or anger. Look at the book of Lamentations: five whole chapters of heartbreak and mourning. And Ecclesiastes chapter 3 says that for *everything* there is a season—a time to mourn and a time to dance.

While some parts of church culture may encourage mourning for only a brief period (like a night or two, but definitely not longer than a month, O ye of little faith!), Scripture tells us that suffering can last a long time. Abraham's wife, Sarah, was barren until age ninety. Joseph was sold into slavery by his brothers and was imprisoned for years. David was anointed as the future king of Israel by Samuel when he was a mere shepherd boy but waited fifteen to twenty years before he actually became king. And David spent most of those years running from King Saul, who was trying to murder him! (Read the book of Psalms and hear his suffering for yourself.)

Perhaps we feel guilty for being sad, even though we know how good God is. Or we feel ashamed of our anger with our circumstances, knowing the immense suffering Jesus endured on the cross for our salvation. Maybe we feel we have no right to question God, wondering who we are—mere humans—to challenge a holy and sovereign God. And perhaps we struggle to voice our pain, whether the physical ache of menstrual suffering or the deeper emotional toll of hormonal imbalances, because it feels insignificant in comparison to what others face. Regardless of why you suppress your real and valid emotions, consider this your permission to be angry, hurt, disappointed, and frustrated. As your sister in Christ, I need to tell you that God isn't scared of your feelings. Better yet, He already knows your thoughts before you say them, so there's nothing you can say that would shock Him, make Him look at you differently, or love you any less. He created you in *His* image, meaning that all of the emotions you feel, He feels tenfold.

Remember the story of Jesus's dear friend Lazarus? Lazarus had two sisters, Mary and Martha, and they all lived in a town called Bethany. Lazarus fell sick, and his sisters sent word to Jesus to let Him know that things weren't looking good. Instead of leaving right then and there, He waited two extra days to visit Lazarus (Jesus knew all along that He would bring him back to life for the purpose of revealing God's glory). Well, within those days, Lazarus died. When Jesus and the disciples made it to Bethany, Lazarus had already been in his grave for four days. Martha ran out to Jesus exclaiming that if He had been there a few days sooner, her brother wouldn't have died. Shortly after, Mary came to Jesus and fell at his feet weeping, expressing the same disappointment as her sister. John 11:33 tells us, "When Jesus saw her weeping, and the Jews who had come along with her also weeping, he was deeply moved in spirit and troubled."

Here we see a man who is fully God and fully human moved so deeply that He was troubled. Verse 35 goes on to say that Jesus wept. Full-on, chest-wheezing, snot-bubbling sobs. Okay, I don't know that for sure, but I can imagine that's how Jesus mourns when we mourn.

The part of the story that stands out to me is that Mary and Martha were left to lament for the better part of a week before Jesus came. They sobbed, heartbroken and hopeless. They questioned why Jesus didn't come sooner, maybe even feeling resentful knowing that He could have prevented their brother's death.

Mary and Martha sat in their suffering.

But Jesus didn't abandon them. He mourned with them.

And then He raised Lazarus from the dead.

So when you're cycling each month and the pain becomes unbearable, or when you're consumed by other forms of physical suffering, go ahead and be mad. Be disappointed. Press your forehead to the floor as your tears stain the carpet. Be so upset that you have no other choice than to scream out, "Why, God, why?" Don't hold back. You can break down, but the key is to break down *in His presence*. If our earthly parents' hearts break when we go through a difficult time, how much more does our heavenly Father's heart break? And yet, unlike anyone else, He doesn't just watch from a distance—He enters in. He weeps with you, carries what you cannot carry, and promises that even in your weakest place, His strength is made perfect (2 Corinthians 12:9.)

LET IT PRUNE YOU

When I hit a breaking point last year over my never-ending health complications, I heard the Holy Spirit say, "You can let this consume you, or you can let it prune you. All I'm asking is for you to be faithful."

That message hit the depths of my soul.

Even if we can't change our circumstances, we can change our mindset. Perception can shape our reality. What I've learned over the years is that suffering is the place where we are pruned, purified, and sanctified. We so badly want to pray away our difficult season, and rightfully so—sometimes the pain is so unbearable that we'd do anything to remove the hurt—but it's in the most painful pit moments that God does something beautiful in you if you let Him.

Instead of asking God to take you out, ask Him what He's trying to do *in* you.

I'm not saying you need a cancer scare or a life-changing diagnosis to be refined. What I am saying is that every challenge we face is an opportunity to allow God to make us look more like His Son. When our hormones shift, when our PMS bubbles up inside us, when situations arise that put a strain on our health, we're reminded of just how human we are and how desperately we need to rely on the Lord to get us through. And the gift that we receive in the end is a stronger faith and a better appreciation of our womanhood.

Jesus says in John 16:33, "I have told you these things, so that in me you may have peace. In this world you will have trouble. But take heart! I have overcome the world." What an incredible promise He makes to us—that regardless of the suffering we endure on this side of creation, He has already defeated it. The world can hurt our bodies, but it cannot touch our souls. And one day we'll have perfect heavenly bodies in the new creation, where no affliction or pain can reach us. What good news we have in Jesus!

I feel you so deeply, my friend. I hope you know how badly I'd like to sit beside you, give you a hug, and sob together about how hard life can be and how painful our periods can be. But God is inviting you to experience His goodness as He turns your mourning into dancing. Whether you're dealing with period cramps, infertility, loss—whatever mountain you're currently looking up at with a discouraged heart—sister, you are perfectly positioned for a miracle.

And the miracle doesn't have to be physical healing; sometimes the greatest miracle is a renewed mind and joy amid the suffering. It's truly divine that in the middle of our furnace of suffering, we can laugh and experience overwhelming, unexplainable peace. Who else besides Jesus can calm the raging storm with three words: "Peace! Be still!"

That's the God we serve.

Be real with Him and let Him shelter you under His wings. Praise Him through the pain. Give thanks amid the trial.

If God is allowing you to endure suffering, then let your suffering give Him glory.

PRACTICAL APPLICATION

- The next time you're overwhelmed with negative thoughts, perhaps while awaiting a test result, speak God's truth out loud. Jeremiah 29:11 is a good verse to start with: "'For I know the plans I have for you,' declares the LORD, 'plans to prosper you and not to harm you, plans to give you hope and a future.'"
- Journal every day for a week. Getting your thoughts and emotions down on paper is not only a great release for your brain but also a special way to connect with the Lord.

- Confide in a friend, family member, or mentor. Honesty and vulnerability allow you to offload the weight you've been carrying. The loving-kindness from your community is healing and biblical!

SCRIPTURE TO MEDITATE ON

- "I have told you these things, so that in me you may have peace. In this world you will have trouble. But take heart! I have overcome the world." (John 16:33)
- "'For I know the plans I have for you,' declares the Lord, 'plans to prosper you and not to harm you, plans to give you hope and a future.'" (Jeremiah 29:11)

SIX

TEN THINGS EVERY WOMAN SHOULD KNOW ABOUT HER HORMONES

MY BEST FRIEND, NICOLE, SAT ON THE COUCH WITH ME ONE DAY and asked me to explain everything I knew about hormone and menstrual health.

"What do you want to know in particular?" I asked. She replied, "Everything. I know nothing."

At first I was surprised, but then I remembered that I too knew zilch about hormone health a few years ago. I had to dig to find information because the extent of my sexual education in middle school was *Don't have sex before marriage or you'll go to hell.* Nothing about how periods work, what happens in puberty, or why I was experiencing the wildest mood swings. If you can relate to this, I apologize on behalf of the schooling system. But what blew Nicole's mind was not that there are four phases of the menstrual cycle but that everything we touch, ingest, smell, put on our skin, and wear has an impact on our health.

I could write an entire separate book listing everything women should know about their health, but I've narrowed it down to my top ten must-knows. Each holds equal significance, and they are presented in no particular order.

Let's begin!

1. Your hormones do more than give you a period.

Hormones—chemical messengers that travel all throughout your body via the bloodstream—have more jobs than simply making you bleed each month. As you've learned, hormones regulate various vital processes in your body, including metabolism, stress management, sleep, growth, and reproduction. They are crucial for maintaining homeostasis (balance) in your body to keep physiological processes running optimally! And there are different types: sex hormones (like estrogen and progesterone), thyroid and metabolism hormones (like T3 and T4), adrenal gland hormones (like cortisol and adrenaline), pancreatic hormones (like insulin), and others (like oxytocin and melatonin). All of these hormones work in harmony to keep you running at your very best. They do more for your body than you can imagine!

2. The environment you live in can make it difficult for your body to thrive.

Our ancestors had a leg up on us in the department of holistic health. Back in the day, there weren't as many toxins in our air or genetically modified foods, hormone-injected animals, synthetic chemicals in beauty and cleaning products, or crops sprayed with pesticides and herbicides. Processed foods have been around for a while, but it wasn't until the 1980s that ultra-processed foods started flooding the grocery stores.[1] High-fructose corn syrup became a staple in sodas, and snacks became drenched in seed oils (vegetable, sunflower, soybean, canola). The worst part is, advertisements made us believe these ingredients were good for us!

Aside from food, the makeup and skincare products you use, the perfume you spray on yourself, and even the shampoo you lather onto your scalp can contain toxic chemicals such as parabens and phthalates—synthetic chemicals that mimic estrogen in the body and have been scientifically proven to disrupt the endocrine system.[2] We'll take a closer look at these chemicals in chapter 9, where you'll learn what ingredients to avoid when shopping for everyday products.

Escaping these endocrine-disrupting chemicals is nearly impossible; they're everywhere. So don't be discouraged if you're trying to live a nontoxic life but can't seem to do it to perfection; nobody can unless they're living off the land in the middle of nowhere. Do your sustainable best. The most important thing is being aware of these harmful chemicals and additives and giving yourself the grace to partner with the Lord in becoming a holier and healthier you.

3. Overconsumption of caffeine can work against your hormones.

Caffeine is more than an addictive substance; it can disrupt your hormones, including insulin, cortisol, and reproductive hormones, for hours after you drink it. It also influences blood sugar and, of course, sleep. (I'm sorry, caffeine lovers!) I've never been bitten by the coffee bug, but every time I do drink it, my anxiety shoots through the roof, my hands get shaky, and I become hyperemotional. Studies have shown that caffeine increases cortisol (the stress hormone) in women and can even increase the risk of infertility and miscarriage.[3] The pros and cons of coffee are debated heavily and often, but in my opinion, you're better off minimizing your intake. None of this is to instill fear but to provide education and awareness so you can make informed decisions for your unique health.

Here's what happens when you drink caffeine:

1. Caffeine travels through your system, blocking adenosine receptors in the brain. Adenosine is a neurotransmitter that promotes relaxation and sleepiness, so its blockage has a stimulating effect, making you feel more alert and awake.
2. The blockage indirectly activates the sympathetic nervous system—your fight-or-flight response system—signaling the adrenal glands to produce cortisol.
3. Cortisol is produced, increasing your alertness, raising blood sugar levels, and helping your body deal with stress (in the short term).
4. When caffeine is consumed on an empty stomach, cortisol levels can spike because your body perceives the stimulant as a stressor.

Consuming caffeine in excess—typically more than two hundred milligrams a day over long periods—can place a heavy burden on your adrenal glands. Over time, this constant stimulation may leave your stress response system exhausted and struggling to function at its best. I'm not saying to drop caffeine altogether (but if you're inspired, kudos to you!); what I am suggesting is that you track how many cups you drink a day and monitor your everyday activities, like sleep, to watch for any abnormalities. It also wouldn't hurt to test your stress: Try going caffeine-free for a week and see if your anxiety, stress, digestion, and sleep have improved.

4. Blue light from phones and TVs disrupts one of your body's most important functions: sleep.

Sleep is massively underrated. Did you know your immune system works the night shift to clear out any leftover junk while you're dreaming? According to Yale School of Medicine's Dr. Yvonne Chu, "Studies have shown that those who chronically get less than seven hours of sleep a night are three times as likely to develop the common cold compared to those who routinely get eight hours or more of sleep."[4] So what's one of the biggest disruptions to a restorative, healthy sleep? Blue light. Our bodies naturally follow a twenty-four-hour circadian rhythm, where light from the sun signals the brain to be alert and awake, and dark signals it to wind down and rest. In a world where we can flip a switch and have light in darkness, and where our electronic devices become our favorite relaxation methods, our brains get confused.

Melatonin, also known as the sleepy hormone, is secreted from the pituitary gland in the brain. Melatonin production begins soon after it's dark, then peaks between

2:00 and 4:00 a.m. When your body is functioning according to its natural rhythm, sunlight during the day boosts serotonin, which your body later converts into melatonin at night—supporting optimal hormone production. When you keep overhead LED lights on in your house at night, your brain thinks it's still daytime. Scrolling on your phone right before bed has the same effect. Simple, healthy rhythms can go a long way in setting you up for restorative sleep. Try winding down with blue light–blocking glasses in the evening and swapping harsh overhead lights for soft amber, red, or yellow lamps that signal to your body that it's time to rest. Spend fifteen to twenty minutes reading before bed—bonus if it's time in God's Word—and aim for seven to eight hours of sleep in a cool, dark room. These small practices create an environment where both your body and soul can truly recharge.

5. What you eat matters.

In a world that prioritizes convenience over nourishment, it's easy to drift away from God's design for food to be healing and life-giving. Because of our unique hormonal design, women's bodies can be more sensitive to things like blood sugar fluctuations, inflammation, and stress. Conditions like PCOS, for example, often involve insulin resistance, which can make managing your energy and weight more challenging. The good news is, awareness is powerful! Knowing how your body works can help you choose foods that nourish you rather than deplete you. Food is a beautiful gift from God, created to bring healing and provision.

Psalm 104:14–15 says,

> He makes grass grow for the cattle,
> and plants for people to cultivate—
> bringing forth food from the earth:
> wine that gladdens human hearts,
> oil to make their faces shine,
> and bread that sustains their hearts.

Every bite you take is an opportunity to partner with the way God designed your body to bring it into balance, calm inflammation, and create steady energy. Choosing whole, nourishing foods like clean proteins, healthy fats, vibrant fruits, and fiber-rich veggies whenever possible gives your body everything it needs to thrive. But remember: grace first, always. You don't have to eat perfectly to honor your body; you just have to notice what helps you feel more stable and what seems to slow you down. The right meals won't solve every hormonal issue, but they often open the door for healing.

We'll explore diet more in depth in chapter 9, where I share comprehensive lists of hormone-balancing foods for each phase of your cycle.

6. Daily movement is essential.

Movement can look different to every woman depending on personal goals, mobility, and current life situation. That's why I like to say movement is a lifestyle. It can range from exercising at the gym or doing at-home workouts, to going on hikes, to opting for the stairs over the elevator. Every time you break a sweat or make the conscious decision to move your body, you're helping your hormones.

Movement benefits your hormones in the following ways:

- Regulates blood sugar and insulin sensitivity
- Reduces the stress hormones cortisol and adrenaline
- Boosts mood-enhancing hormones like dopamine, serotonin, and endorphins
- Supports thyroid function and metabolic health
- Balances sex hormones like estrogen and progesterone
- Improves sleep quality

As someone who had an unhealthy relationship with working out, I know this area can be difficult to navigate. I want to encourage you to exercise because you want to, not because you have to. When exercise becomes a chore, it sucks out all the fun and reward and becomes a tool the devil will use against you, binding you to shame and guilt. And daily movement doesn't have to be high-intensity interval training seven times a week (this actually strains your hormones; please don't overdo it); it can be taking two fifteen-minute walks during your day. If you're doing something each day to get your blood flowing and muscles working, your hormones will thank you.

7. Less is more.

Women have a gift from God that the enemy sometimes uses as a curse: a desire to make sure everyone is taken care of and provided for that often leaves too little time for self-care. Some people call it people-pleasing, but I believe it's a God-given gift that makes women incredible nurturers. It's part of our maternal code, but failing to take time to slow down can be the downfall of our health. Our hormones can handle a lot, but only to a certain point. When you go, go, go without stopping, your cortisol production goes through the roof, putting extreme strain on your adrenal glands (the glands that produce stress hormones). Imagine there's an alarm bell in your body that never shuts off. The hypothalamic-pituitary-adrenal (HPA) axis is the system that regulates this alarm. When it has had enough, it will let you know. Eventually, your body becomes so tired of keeping up with the sounding alarm that it burns out, leading to chronic fatigue, brain fog, low blood sugar, depression, and gut issues.

I give you permission to take things slowly: Walk slower in public places, savoring the moment instead of rushing from one thing to the next. Turn off any background noise when you're cooking at home, and stop pushing yourself too hard in the gym, at work, and in your family life. You deserve to be taken care of, and your body deserves a break. The same God who built sabbath into the week built pauses into your body, reminding you that slowing down is not weakness but wisdom.

8. Your periods shouldn't be debilitating.

This one blew my mind: Though PMS is common, it can be a sign that there are underlying issues. Every woman is different and reacts in a unique way, and some women have never experienced PMS! I'm jealous! Though I too have experienced painless periods through experimenting with cycle syncing—making food, exercise, and lifestyle choices that align with your hormones throughout your cycle. Granted, it's a lot of effort and requires intentionality, but it is possible.

If you suffer from PMS symptoms like mild discomfort or sensations in the uterus, these are common reactions to fluctuating hormones that deserve attention but aren't what I would consider immediate red flags. But if you experience intense pain in your uterus, excruciating cramps, extreme fatigue, and other severe symptoms like suicidal thoughts, it's imperative you speak to a professional. Your period shouldn't make you skip school, call in to work, or cancel plans. And it shouldn't leave you in the fetal position next to the toilet. Finding the right doctor is equally as important because unfortunately a lot of practitioners will tell you either that your severe symptoms are completely normal or all in your head. But just because something is common doesn't mean it's normal. You deserve to be seen, heard, and given the right tools to help ease your period pain.

9. Balanced blood sugar makes the world go round.

If you're like me, you've probably associated the words *blood sugar* with diabetes or high-sugar foods without drawing connections to any other function of the body. But balanced blood sugar is the remedy to a lot of health issues, from metabolic syndrome to PCOS, mood stability, heart health, and hormone health. I'd argue this is one of the most important points, so go ahead and take notes.

Blood sugar (glucose) is the fuel that keeps our cells alive and functioning. Glucose comes from carbohydrates like refined flour (pastas, sweet treats), table sugar, complex carbohydrates (sweet potatoes, barley), and fruit. It's essential for our bodies, but having too much of it can lead to complications.

Blood sugar levels are affected by diet, activity levels,

stress, your microbiome (the bacteria in the gut), and body fat. When glucose enters the bloodstream, the pancreas is alerted to release insulin. Insulin is an important hormone that allows cells to use glucose for energy or storage. You can think of insulin as the key that unlocks the door to your cells. When there's a glucose overload, like when you eat a carb-heavy meal, insulin can't always keep up. When that happens, your cells become overcrowded and don't let glucose in, so it lingers in your bloodstream, raising blood sugar levels, resulting in increased blood pressure and inflammation. You may have experienced this when you had a hearty bowl of pasta and an hour or two later your heart was racing.

So why would this be an issue for your hormones? Over time, your cells become so overcrowded that new influxes of glucose can be rejected, becoming stored in the body as visceral fat, particularly around the abdomen. Visceral fat contains an enzyme called aromatase that converts androgens (like testosterone) into estrogen. This process is called aromatization.[5] If you already struggle with estrogen dominance, like PCOS, then the more visceral fat you have, the more estrogen is likely to be produced. The ovaries also have insulin receptors. Excess insulin can cause them to make testosterone rather than their usual estrogen and progesterone. Do you see how this hamster wheel keeps spinning?

The good news is that there are simple ways to control blood sugar levels, which we'll get to later.

10. You're not stuck forever.

God is in the business of making a way where there is no way, and His healing touch has not vanished. If you suffer from endometriosis, ovarian cysts, PCOS, hypothyroidism,

PMDD, or pain of any kind, you're not stuck. I've watched God shrink lymph nodes in my body and have witnessed cysts disappear in others, but the greatest miracles I've witnessed are when women befriend their ailments and learn to see the beauty within the struggle. I think of my best friend, who was born with cerebral palsy and has walked with a limp her entire life. I've watched her go from hating how God made her to seeing her disability as her superpower. It has become her ministry and life purpose to speak life and hope into others, regardless of their circumstances. She may not be physically healed, but her heart has been radically transformed. That's the kind of healing God offers—a wholeness that goes beyond what the eye can see.

Maybe God is writing your testimony at this very moment, amid the pain and frustration. I may not know the outcome of your situation, but I know that our God weeps when we weep and grieves when we feel hopeless. So I'm standing with you in faith, praying for your physical healing, but even more than that, I pray for your heart to be transformed and for your mind to be renewed. I declare in Jesus's name that no weapon formed against you will prosper! Don't lose hope when you find yourself in a valley. What feels impossible is possible for God. Continue to pray and praise Him through it all.

As you've learned, hormones play a larger role than simply giving you a period. They are the backbone of your health and work together to keep you at your healthiest. The good news is that through simple lifestyle changes paired with prayer and Scripture, healing can be found, and your hormones can find balance once again. Take courage from these ten insights about hormones, and know that your body is working endlessly to keep you balanced. Whether your current focus is a healthy diet, exercise, adequate sleep, or less time scrolling social media, each step you take helps support your health. And as you go throughout your week, try implementing one or more of the following hormone-friendly lifestyle suggestions.

PRACTICAL APPLICATION

→ Swap screen time before bed for thirty minutes of Bible reading.
→ Turn off overhead lights at night and utilize lamps with warm lighting.
→ Say no to an obligation or task that has been giving you anxiety.
→ Go for two fifteen-minute walks daily for the next seven days.
→ Instead of drinking coffee on an empty stomach, try matcha or another type of tea after breakfast.

SCRIPTURE TO MEDITATE ON

→ "He makes grass grow for the cattle, and plants for people to cultivate—bringing forth food from the earth: wine that gladdens human hearts, oil to make their faces shine, and bread that sustains their hearts." (Psalm 104:14–15)

SEVEN

YOUR BODY IS A TEMPLE. SERIOUSLY.

IF SOMEONE FOLLOWED YOU AROUND FOR A WEEK AND TRACKED what you ate, what you drank, how much you moved, how much you slept, and how you handled stress, what would the final report say? Would you walk away feeling encouraged and inspired, or would you be challenged to make some changes? Scripture reminds us that our bodies are temples of the Holy Spirit (1 Corinthians 6:19–20), yet many of us (me included!) treat them more like convenience stores—quick and easy, cluttered, and filled with things that don't truly nourish. Instead of intentionally fueling our bodies, we tend to grab whatever's convenient because of the busyness, the parenting, the schoolwork, the job demands, the ministry, and the list goes on. I know I've been guilty of grabbing what's easy instead of what's best.

But stewardship is a privilege. Stewardship asks, "What

am I doing with what I've been given?" God has gifted us with bodies that fight to keep us healthy, strong, and alert. And for women, our bodies give us the opportunity to bring new life into the world. Our bodies are sacred real estate, the very place the Holy Spirit dwells. If that doesn't prove your worth, then I don't know what will.

Christians often separate the physical from the spiritual. Some people believe that focusing on rest, nutrition, and movement is selfish or even vain. But I'm here to cast that lie right back where it came from in Jesus's name because God cares about your entire being—mind, body, soul, and spirit. And let me remind you that Jesus lived on this earth in a body; He wasn't a ghostlike figure or phantom spirit. He occupied a body, just like you and me. He laid His physical hands on people, spoke bold and redemptive words with His physical voice, and was physically present. So while caring for our spirits is essential, pouring into our God-given vessel is important too.

First Corinthians 6:19–20 says, "Do you not know that your bodies are temples of the Holy Spirit, who is in you, whom you have received from God? You are not your own; you were bought at a price. Therefore honor God with your bodies." The Greek word translated "temple" in this verse refers to the physical holy sanctuary where God dwelled before Jesus came to earth. The book of Exodus portrays the Israelites' journey out of slavery in Egypt. But they hit a few bumps on the road to freedom. They questioned God's goodness and Moses's leadership and often tried to take matters into their own hands. They particularly had a knack for creating idols, even though they were forbidden to make any objects or images to represent God (Exodus 20:4–5). However, God recognized their humanity and honored their desire for something physical and visual, so He gave them the tabernacle. This was a tent that served as a mobile temple, which was later replaced by the temple in Jerusalem.

The tabernacle was divided into three chambers: the outer court, the Holy Place, and the Most Holy Place—or holy of holies. The word *holy* at its most basic level means "set apart" or "different."[1] This is significant because holiness is what set Yahweh apart from pagan gods. He is also set apart from sin since He is perfect in all ways. The Holy Place and the Most Holy Place were set apart because God was present there.

The outer court served as the grounds for sacrificial guilt and sin offerings, and in the middle was a tent that only the priests could enter—because it was, you guessed it, holy. The tabernacle had one entrance that led straight into the second chamber, the Holy Place. In it were three pieces of furniture: a golden lampstand, the table for the bread of presence, and the altar of incense. Fun fact: Jesus used these symbols to show He is God by saying He is the light of the world (John 8:12) and the bread of life (John 6:35). The third chamber, the Most Holy Place, was a smaller room housing the ark of the covenant. This chamber could be entered only once a year, by the high priest on the Day of Atonement, and only with a blood sacrifice.

When Jesus died on the cross, the curtain between the temple's Holy Place and Most Holy Place tore from top to bottom (Matthew 27:51), symbolizing that the way to God was now open to anyone and everyone through Jesus. The blood of an animal was no longer needed to atone for sin; the sacrificial Lamb Himself shed His blood once and for all, washing the world's sins away. Hebrews 10:19–20 (NLT) says, "Dear brothers and sisters, we can boldly enter heaven's Most Holy Place because of the blood of Jesus. By his death, Jesus opened a new and life-giving way through the curtain into the Most Holy Place."

I think about the woman with the issue of blood, those riddled with disease and infirmities, the women on the outskirts of town on their periods—all those forbidden from temple worship—running into the arms of Jesus. I think about the countless women who have messaged me sharing their miscarriage grief, infertility struggles, and loss. I think of the young girls around the world getting their period for the first time, afraid and confused with no one to turn to. I think about you and me, carrying the weight of life, being wrapped in His loving embrace. What Jesus did on the cross gave heartbroken people like us a nonrefundable ticket to everlasting life with Him.

THE TEMPLE IS YOU

Maybe you're reading this with tears in your eyes (I'm teary as I write this) because it's hard to wrap your head around the fact that God loves you so much that He chose you and me to be temples of His presence. And if God meant to convey the idea that the Spirit lives within the believer in a blasé way, He could've used a word like *residence* or *house*, but He chose *temple* because we are much more than just a house to Him. Therefore, everything we do—how we act, speak, and think and what we let into our heart and mind—matters. It's an undeserved honor that we get to nurture the Spirit of God, but with this honor comes responsibility and intentionality.

Each person's relationship with the Lord is unique and special, so the way you steward your temple may look a little different from the way someone else's does. Maybe you have no idea where to start, what to change, or how to even begin this stewarding journey. I encourage you to pause and reflect on all that God has entrusted to you—your body that works tirelessly to keep you healthy, your willing spirit, your servant heart—and ask yourself, "Am I using these gifts in a way that aligns with God's will and glorifies Him?"

Ask yourself these questions and answer honestly:

- → Does the food I eat honor the body God gave me, or can I grow in the area of nutrition to help my body thrive?
- → Do I push myself to be in good physical health (regardless of weight)?
- → Do I give myself permission to say no and slow down so I can prioritize rest?
- → Do I acknowledge my period pain and hormonal symptoms, or do I gaslight myself into believing they're not a big deal?
- → Am I taking tangible action steps to help alleviate my hormone-related symptoms?
- → Have I been asking God or others for help?

The best first step is acknowledging your desire to honor God with your body. I can offer all kinds of advice to help you balance your hormones, alleviate your pain, and choose great food to bring relief, but if you don't feel the conviction and the readiness to put that advice into practice, you'll remain on the hormonal hamster wheel. And it's okay if you're not ready yet; this is a lifelong journey. The most amazing news is that you're not doing this in your own strength; it's God who's directing your path and cheering you on every step of the way. You may take one step forward and two steps back, but it doesn't matter because the lover of your soul is so proud that you want to take steps in the first place.

My hope is that these words stirred something deeper within you, a conviction rooted in love. I'm not here to judge or point a finger; I couldn't if I tried. Lord knows I'd be the biggest hypocrite! I'm right here with you—learning, unlearning, stepping out of comfort zones, and choosing daily to pick up my cross and follow Him. We're in this together, running the race side by side, committed to stewarding this sacred gift of life as we give ourselves grace to grow and show a willingness to be sanctified.

PRACTICAL APPLICATION

→ As you go throughout your week, mark anything you've done to grow in the areas of physical, emotional, or spiritual health.

BODY-AS-A-TEMPLE TRACKER

DAY	PHYSICAL	EMOTIONAL	SPIRITUAL
Sunday			
Monday			
Tuesday			
Wednesday			
Thursday			
Friday			
Saturday			

SCRIPTURE TO MEDITATE ON

- "Do you not know that your bodies are temples of the Holy Spirit, who is in you, whom you have received from God? You are not your own; you were bought at a price. Therefore honor God with your bodies." (1 Corinthians 6:19–20)
- "Dear brothers and sisters, we can boldly enter heaven's Most Holy Place because of the blood of Jesus. By his death, Jesus opened a new and life-giving way through the curtain into the Most Holy Place." (Hebrews 10:19–20 NLT)

EIGHT

MORE THAN A BABY MAKER

***Disclaimer: This chapter covers infertility, miscarriage, and other sensitive topics. Read with a guarded heart and know that Jesus is wrapping His loving arms around you. If this material is too much at the moment, feel free to skip it.**

"I'M SO SORRY, I CAN'T FIND A HEARTBEAT."

These are words every pregnant woman is terrified to hear. Words that scar. Few heartbreaks are more invisible than the ones carried in silence and isolation: the negative tests, the disappointment when your period arrives, the nursery that stays vacant. Infertility, loss, miscarriage—they don't just affect the body and mind. Your identity and worth can feel shaken, and that screams a louder message: *What's wrong with me?*

A million questions race through your mind as the future that you wanted so desperately isn't looking anything like you hoped and prayed for. Your dreams and faith take a massive blow. The waiting feels like a hopeless infinity, and the healing process feels hurtful.

If I can't have a baby, what does that make me?

It's not spoken out loud in church, but somewhere along the way, we started believing the lie that a woman's worth is measured by her womb, that motherhood is the ultimate marker of purpose, and that the main way God will use us is by our staying home and raising children. But what happens if the baby doesn't come? Or comes but is lost too soon? What about the women who have tried year after year, spending thousands of dollars for their prayers to be answered? What about the women who have lost their children? Or the ones who can't bear to try again for fear of another heartbreak? And what about the women who do not desire to have kids at all?

I used to think I had the right words for women walking through these different scenarios. But the more I sat with the stories, the more I learned to simply *listen*. Because there's a depth to each kind of loss that I may never be able to understand, and words can't fix it. The pain and grief run deep over what has been taken and what has never been given. Shame, anger, and frustration arise as you shake your fist at God for giving you what feels like a broken body. And beneath it all you can't even seem to find where God is in all of this.

If God is so good, why did He let this happen?

If that's your question, if you're carrying a heavy burden or quiet anger, I want you to know that you're not broken. And you're certainly not less of a woman. The best thing about God is that He doesn't define your worth by anything other than simply being His. And He promises to work everything out for good. I'm not going to sit here and throw verse after verse at you in hopes of miraculously making all the pain go away (I'm sure there are plenty of people in your life already doing so), but I will give you the space to be angry, frustrated, confused, sad, and hurt. I will be right here with you as your tears spill onto these pages.

Throughout this chapter you will read stories from women who have walked in your shoes. These are real women who have wrestled with infertility, miscarriage, grief, confusion, and waiting. Their journey may not look exactly like yours, and their ending may not be the same as what God has for you. But their pain and longing will feel familiar. Some of their stories end in miracles, some end with unexplainable peace despite their circumstances, and others are still unfolding. May their resilience remind you that God is not done with you yet.

You'll also hear from my personal OB/GYN, Dr. John Lundberg—who delivered me from my mother's womb—on how he helps couples struggling with infertility, heartbreak, and a lost sense of purpose. Dr. Lundberg is a wise and deeply trusted man of God. As an elder at his church in New Jersey and a seasoned physician with over thirty years of experience, he's walked closely with me through some of the most difficult moments of my health and faith. He's held my hand and prayed with me, standing in faith alongside me as I faced frightening diagnoses and underwent reproductive procedures.

The stories you're about to read are tender and honest. In their vulnerability, you may hear whispers of your own story. I invite you to enter them with compassion and an open heart.

Hannah, 30

I was never the girl who couldn't wait to be a mom. I knew I wanted to get married and have kids one day, but for me it was more a step in the process rather than a passion I felt called to. That being said, I never anticipated motherhood and the journey to becoming a mom to be so challenging. My husband and I found out we were going to have our first baby about a year into our marriage—we were so excited! I had some complications during the pregnancy, and my plans went out the window (from unmedicated home birth to a scheduled C-section), but ultimately our son arrived, and he and I were both healthy. It took me a while to find my rhythm in motherhood. I felt like it didn't come naturally to me, and I struggled with that for a long time, but we knew we wanted to have more kids, so we started trying when our son was about eighteen months. I found out I was pregnant a few months later, but days before our son's second birthday, I found out we had lost the baby.

I was shocked. It was so unexpected, especially after carrying my son to term. I never even considered that loss could be a possibility for me. It was extremely traumatic for several reasons.

At my second OB appointment is when we discovered there was no longer a heartbeat, but my body hadn't started the process yet. I chose to wait and see if it would happen naturally, and after thirteen days my body finally started the process.

After this, I had two more miscarriages, and I started to wonder if maybe God didn't want me to have more kids. I already felt insecure about my ability to mother my son and thought I didn't deserve to mother more children. I started getting more honest with God than I ever had. Going through that kind of grief and disappointment brought me face-to-face with a kind of suffering I hadn't experienced in my faith before, but it ended up being the exact thing that made my relationship with God stronger.

I had a dream before my husband and I even met that I would have a son and a daughter one day, so in January 2023 during prayer and fasting at our church, I told God I would try one more time. If I got pregnant again, it would be my fifth pregnancy, so I asked God to either help me conceive or shift my heart to fostering or adoption. The next week, I found out I was pregnant. Shortly after, we found out it was a girl!

Not far into that pregnancy, I started having complications and I was terrified. I developed a ton of conditions and felt so disappointed. I was praying one day and said, "God, I thought this was the redemption story!" And He said, "It is." He reminded me that just because it isn't free of struggle doesn't mean He is no longer good. It wasn't the way I would've chosen, but I held on to that until our daughter was born at thirty-five weeks. I held on to it when she was in the NICU, and I'm still holding on to it today as we approach her second birthday. She is alive and healthy, and so is my relationship with Jesus.

I would never have chosen this journey, and I wish no other

woman ever had to experience it, but God has been so kind to me in the midst of it all.

Through loss, fear, and unmet expectations, Hannah's faith deepened—not because the pain disappeared but because God showed Himself present in it. Even as she questioned His plans, He met her with overwhelming love. Hannah's journey reminds us that redemption often unfolds in the middle of the battle, not after it's over.

Let's continue this journey to hear Destiny's story—one that didn't end the way she expected, but one full of God's faithfulness.

Destiny, 26

I found out I was pregnant just a few weeks after my husband and I had celebrated our honeymoon. The pregnancy was unplanned and not part of what I had envisioned for my life—at least not for a while. I needed a few hours of silence to fully process the reality that I was going to be a mother for the first time. Eventually, I fully accepted and believed that if this was God calling me into motherhood, then I would follow, even though I didn't feel quite ready. Over the next few weeks, my husband and I prepared our lives to welcome a baby girl. However, a persistent fear of miscarriage kept replaying in my mind, over and over. But each time, I reminded myself, "That thought isn't from Jesus—it's just a scare tactic from the Enemy." I kept brushing it off because I truly believed that God had chosen me for this journey into motherhood.

But after reaching thirteen weeks of pregnancy, I started experiencing an uncomfortable pain in my abdomen that persisted for four days. Eventually, the pain was followed by bleeding. My husband and I visited the hospital, and the doctors discharged me after they detected the baby's heartbeat and said there was nothing to worry about. But deep down, I felt that something was still wrong. The next day, the bleeding continued, and my husband and I decided to visit the hospital again. While there, I quickly noticed that the nurses were struggling to find a heartbeat. Then I realized this might be my worst nightmare happening. As I thought about the possibility of our baby not making it, I quickly found myself in prayer. I prayed to God during the one hour of silence while I waited for the doctor to visit my room. I told God, "If our baby girl is in heaven right now, then I have peace knowing she's with you. It's not the outcome I wanted, but as long as Caleb [my husband] and I created a soul that will follow and serve you in heaven, then I'm okay with that." I cried and cried, and then tried to pull myself together, but deep down I felt the need to brace myself for the worst.

Eventually, the doctor entered the room to tell me the news: "Unfortunately, the ultrasound results indicated there was no heartbeat. I'm so sorry. It seems that your body is at the beginning stages of a miscarriage." I started bawling immediately. After some time and discussion, the hospital discharged me so that I could experience the miscarriage naturally at home. For the next three to four hours, I cried, yelled, and crawled in pain in my bathroom, with my husband holding my hand the entire time. It truly felt like labor—it was the worst physical pain I had ever endured in my life. Eventually, my body released what used to be in my uterus, and I yelled and cried out even more because I knew that was our baby girl. I felt my heart shatter into pieces.

Now, almost four weeks later and preparing to celebrate Mother's Day, I still firmly believe that God called me into motherhood. I know without a doubt that God made no mistake when He created my baby girl in my womb. Although I miss her dearly, she gave me a glimpse of what motherhood could be—and it was the most painful but beautiful experience of my life. Although I cried many tears, I thank God for the gift of carrying her for three and a half months. At first, I used to cry because I thought, "Why would God call me into motherhood just to take it away from me?" but over time I saw things differently. God didn't take motherhood away from me—because I am still a mother. I'm a mom to a baby angel in heaven. Just because my baby girl didn't make it to birth doesn't mean I'm not a mother, and it certainly doesn't mean I failed at being one.

During my pregnancy, I prayed every single day for two things: that God would keep both my baby and me safe and that my baby girl would grow up to be a follower of Jesus. Recently, I realized that God answered both of those prayers. We both are safe, and my baby girl gets to follow Jesus for all eternity in heaven. That's more than I ever could have asked for from my first pregnancy, even though the outcome looked different from what I had hoped. Overall, this experience has reminded me of one powerful truth: God is still good, and He is always faithful.

What moved me to tears was Destiny's reaction to the fear that she may have been miscarrying. She cried out to God and surrendered her will and her baby's life into His hands. That type of faith is inspiring. It says, *God, I really don't want this to be true, but if it has to be, I trust You and I have peace knowing that Your will is greater than mine.* Though the

Lord brought her baby girl home to heaven, He gave her peace that surpasses all understanding and the reassurance that no matter the circumstance, He's always faithful.

Now let's hear from Kathryn, whose story shows how God uses His people to be His hands and feet on earth to bring encouragement and prayer support to the brokenhearted.

Kathryn, 31

In March 2023 my husband and I found out we were pregnant; we were flooded with emotions—excitement and joy. It was not planned, but we also weren't preventing it from happening. We eagerly shared the news with our family, and after the first ultrasound, we rushed to our parents and in-laws to show them the picture. Quickly, we began thinking and talking about how different our future would be. After I made it to eight weeks, we had to schedule another appointment to listen to the baby's heartbeat. The appointment was scheduled for the Thursday before Mother's Day. Unfortunately, we never got to hear my baby's heartbeat.

Sunday night, a week before Mother's Day of 2023, I had been spotting, and I knew in my gut something was wrong. I went to the ER alone; my husband is a night shift nurse so he couldn't come. After a few hours and some testing, they couldn't confirm or deny whether I was experiencing a miscarriage. I was sent home, and the miscarriage happened. The miscarriage was the most painful experience both emotionally and physically. I was blessed to have my husband home with me that night. There was nothing he could do but to offer his support. I couldn't believe this was happening. Since the moment I found out I was pregnant, I prayed to God to keep my baby safe because I didn't know what would happen to me if the baby didn't make it. The next day, my sister called me out of the blue to check up on me and the baby, and I had to share the unfortunate news with her. She is also a nurse and told me that, although it was hard, I needed to go to the ER to make sure everything was okay internally.

I can't remember the physician's name, but I wish I could because the words he told me have been etched on my heart forever. The physician told me that there was nothing wrong with my body, it wasn't something I could have controlled, and sometimes this just happens. He shared a bit of his story about how his wife and he had experienced something similar and now had a happy and healthy baby after years of trying, and he was sure I'd be able to share the same story of success.

Sunday was Mother's Day, the first Mother's Day I thought I'd be able to celebrate because I was expecting, but instead of celebrating, we were mourning the loss of our child. Fast-forward a few Sundays: The pastor welcomed anyone who needed prayer to come to the altar. I was guided to a member and told her what had happened—I was really angry with God. I had begged Him not to take my baby away, but He did just that. She prayed over me, and for God to fill me with His comfort, peace, and guidance.

A few days later, I remember kneeling in my bedroom crying and pleading to God to please take the pain and grief because it was too great to bear, and He did! It was like a calmness or peace that washed over me. And since that day I have never been the same—my life has been transformed.

It is May 2025, and I wish I could say I'm pregnant, but I am not. What I can say is my relationship with God has been better than ever. The reason I wanted to share this is because women should know they are not alone. In tragedy we can either seek God or stay stuck. I chose to seek God, and I promise you that is the best thing I could have ever done.

Kathryn's story reminds me of how important the body of Christ is. Each of us has unique giftings that the Lord asks us to use to edify the body of believers. God used her doctor and church community to pour light into a dark place. Through the power of prayer, and with an earnest and seeking heart, Kathryn experienced a breakthrough. It didn't erase what had happened, but it allowed her to see her future with fresh eyes and a renewed spirit. That's our God! He makes broken things beautiful.

This next story is relatable in many ways and addresses a question you may have asked God yourself: "Is it too late?" Let's dive into Donna's testimony.

Donna, 45

My name is Donna, and my journey with infertility has been less about diagnosis and more about unanswered questions. At forty-five, I've never had children. I've been in a long-term relationship with someone who has children from a previous marriage, so I know the opportunity for kids existed. I was on birth control for over a decade for various reasons, and now I find myself wondering, "Was it ever meant to be?" I can't say for certain that I'm infertile, but the silence on this matter has spoken volumes. And now as I navigate perimenopause, there's a lingering weight—the stigma, the assumptions, the quiet grief of time slipping away.

I'm in a transitional season—spiritually, emotionally, and professionally. I lost my job two months ago and have spent most of my life in stressful leadership roles. Truthfully, I don't want to go back to that life. But it was in this stillness, this stripping away of what I thought defined me, that God met me. I didn't grow up with strong faith. For years I felt forgotten, unseen by God—just watching others move forward while I stood still. But when I was forty-four, He flipped the switch. Suddenly, I could see clearly. After years of wandering, I realized God had been pursuing me all along.

I still have so many unanswered questions. I'm unmarried, transitioning careers, rediscovering my identity, and learning how to walk with God through it all. But I believe He has placed a calling on my heart to speak about my journey—for women like me, in seasons like this. You don't have to have it all figured out to be used by God. You just have to say yes.

I hope Donna's story spoke straight to your heart and declared, "It's never too late." No matter what the world wants to label you, God doesn't determine your worth and value based on your age. What pleases God is obedience, no matter what the situation looks like. Job, no job, kids, no kids—God uses it all.

When the world instills fear, God offers something different. Let's look at Aniya's story—one that teaches the importance of listening to your body and trusting God above all else.

Aniya, 27

In 2022, just a few months into a new relationship, I was told something no woman ever wants to hear: "You may not be able to have children."

I had been struggling with PCOS and endometriosis, and the doctors were firm. They handed me prescriptions—birth control and metformin—and sent me on my way. I was devastated. I remember feeling ashamed and embarrassed, especially because my relationship with Omar, who would later become my husband, was still new. I didn't want him to feel like he was signing up for a life of uncertainty.

But his response was simple, steady, and full of faith: "Don't worry. God is in control."

That became my anchor.

I didn't take the medication. I chose a different path—one that felt more in tune with my body and spirit. I focused on healing holistically: movement, nourishing food, and inner peace. For a full year, I poured myself into caring for my body naturally. But the truth is, I still didn't feel great. I was tired, foggy, and unsure if any of it was working.

Then, in spring 2023, something shifted. I felt off—warm and uneasy. On a whim, I took a pregnancy test. Positive. Then another. And another. I took five in total. All positive.

After everything—the fear, the shame, the slow healing, and the waiting—I was pregnant.

In January 2024, I gave birth to my miracle: Ayub. His name means Job in Arabic—a biblical figure known for enduring suffering with unwavering faith.

And that's exactly what he brought into my life: restoration after the storm.

Ayub is proof that healing isn't always linear. That faith can outshine fear. And that miracles come not when we expect them but when we need them most.

Aniya's story makes me want to scream, "That's my God!" What started out as a devastating diagnosis and a temptation to settle for a life defined by limitations became a journey of perseverance. Aniya chose to honor the path of healing she felt was right for her body, and in God's timing, healing bloomed into the greatest gift: her son. And now her son lives as a beacon of hope for restoration.

The last story you're about to read is Romans 8:28 come to life—God uses everything for good for those who love Him and are called according to His purpose. Let's read Kari's story together.

Kari, 35

I've spent the last five years in the trenches of infertility. It's a path I never imagined I'd walk, and one I wouldn't wish on anyone. During that time, I've experienced three miscarriages, all after infertility treatments. One of those losses came after our first IVF transfer, when we were overjoyed to be pregnant with a baby girl—only to find out at an ultrasound that her heartbeat had stopped.

During that IVF cycle, I was going through a Bible study series at my church. I remember feeling both incredibly hopeful and deeply terrified. I experienced the high of seeing a positive test and then the crushing low of hearing that we had lost her.

After that, I made a silent decision: I wasn't going back to the Bible study group. I didn't tell anyone, not even my leader. I didn't think I could keep showing up. In fact, I wasn't sure I could keep showing up for God. I felt abandoned, broken, and angry. I didn't want to worship. I didn't want to pray. I didn't want to pretend I was okay.

That weekend, my church hosted a big event tied to the study I was going through. I had zero plans of going. But partway through, my study leader texted me: "It's still not too late . . . I think you should come." I almost ignored it. But then I had this very clear realization: *The Enemy doesn't want me to go.*

So I went.

And that weekend changed everything.

God met me there in my grief. Not with answers. Not with guarantees. But with peace. With presence. With the kind of love that doesn't always remove the pain but sits in it with you.

Now, months later, my relationship with the Lord is stronger than it's ever been. I'm planning to lead the same Bible study this fall. I'm enrolling in a two-year program to deepen my faith. And, most surprising of all, I'm okay with the idea that I may never be a mom in the traditional sense. That doesn't mean the grief is gone. But I've finally fully surrendered. And in that surrender, I've found freedom.

Surrendering to the Lord is one of the most difficult, humbling, and painful things to do as you think about your God-given embodiment. But God doesn't just leave you in your pain; He gives you something in exchange: peace, hope, a renewed spirit, purpose, and joy that no circumstance can steal. When you lay down your will at His feet, He lifts you up with His, reminding you that His plans and ways are greater than your own.

FERTILITY IS NOT YOUR IDENTITY

After hearing the pain, the hope, the redemption, and the raw faith woven through these women's stories, I sat down with Dr. John Lundberg, a board-certified OB/GYN (my OB!) and bold follower of Christ.

When we spoke, he told me how he navigates the heartbreaking experience of miscarriage, loss, and infertility and how he responds to women who say, "Why would God let this happen?" He said, "I always tell them (lovingly) that I'm not God. Because whenever you answer a 'Why God' question, you're taking the place of God and I'm not God. I face tragedy every day. I watch two-year-olds die of cancer and deliver stillborn births, and for me to try to give a quick answer to that or to try to explain it away is cold and not very caring. When it comes to women who can't get pregnant (which I see often) or women who can't find the right man, I say to them, 'I'm sorry for what you're going through.' But I always tell them that God used the prophet Jeremiah mightily, and yet He told him he couldn't get married. Many people in the Bible struggled with fertility issues. And He used them mightily. We pray for what we want. But prayer is supposed to be aligning our wills to God's will. So sometimes God's answer to our prayer is no—not harshly, but because He knows the full course of our lives. We must trust Him in that. Because He's all-good and all-loving and all-knowing and sovereign and providential, I trust that."

NOT MY WILL BUT YOURS

Sometimes our plans and thoughts don't match God's, and when the outcome looks nothing like what we prayed for, it cuts deep. It shakes our faith. In the middle of the heartbreak, Isaiah 55:8–9 provides a lot of comfort:

> "My thoughts are not your thoughts,
> neither are your ways my ways,"
> declares the LORD.
> "As the heavens are higher than the earth,
> so are my ways higher than your ways
> and my thoughts than your thoughts."

We can rest assured that we are right in the palm of His hand and trust that the story He's writing is far greater than what we'd write for ourselves.

Stories like the ones you read earlier remind us that God's presence and mighty hand are woven into every detail, even the ones we can't see. But we can't get too caught up in what God *does*, because most important is *who we are in Him*. Especially in seasons of grief, waiting, or unanswered prayers, our identity can be shaken. Yet the everlasting truth is that your worth is not measured by the status of your womb, what your body can or can't do, a diagnosis, or an outcome. It's rooted in the unchanging, unshakable identity God has spoken over you from the very beginning.

Infertility, loss, miscarriage—it's a wilderness no one chooses but also a place where God is present. Your body may feel broken, your will may feel crushed, but your identity as a daughter of Christ remains intact. Never forget that your body is a holy temple, one bought with a high price. Jesus saw all your brokenness, grief, and sorrow and took it with Him to the cross. You're not defined by what your womb holds but by *who holds you*. And nothing can separate you from His love. Remember Job from the Bible? Everything Job ever loved and cared about was taken away from him. Yet he remained faithful, and God restored all that was taken. And King David was under attack for years and years before he ever saw the throne. But God used all of the hardship they faced for their good.

I don't know what needs to be resurrected in you—hope, joy, peace—but I'm believing that God planted a few seeds in your heart today. I am standing in agreement with the hope found in Christ Jesus; emptiness is not your portion, and fear is not your future. Through the aches and pains our cycles can bring—and the betrayal we can feel from our bodies—He is still sovereign. In the mighty name of Jesus, I declare that restoration is coming and that His peace will take the place in your heart where sorrow once sat. God has never taken His eyes off you. What is now a trial will soon be your greatest testimony!

PRACTICAL APPLICATION

- Give yourself permission to feel grief, anger, or confusion. Bring these emotions to God in prayer, trusting that He will meet you in your pain with love and understanding.
- Surround yourself with trusted friends, mentors, or a faith-based community who can pray with you, listen, and offer encouragement during difficult seasons.
- Remind yourself that your identity is not tied to your circumstances or body but is rooted in being a beloved daughter of Christ.
- Trust that God's ways are higher than ours, even when the outcome doesn't match your hopes. Lean into His sovereignty and faithfulness.
- Reflect on stories of others who have walked similar paths, drawing strength from their resilience and the ways God worked through their trials.

SCRIPTURE TO MEDITATE ON

- "My thoughts are not your thoughts, neither are your ways my ways," declares the Lord. "As the heavens are higher than the earth, so are my ways higher than your ways and my thoughts than your thoughts." (Isaiah 55:8–9)
- "Three times I pleaded with the Lord to take it away from me. But he said to me, 'My grace is sufficient

for you, for my power is made perfect in weakness.' Therefore I will boast all the more gladly about my weaknesses, so that Christ's power may rest on me." (2 Corinthians 12:8–9)

PART THREE

A PACE OF PEACE

NINE

A BIBLICAL APPROACH TO CYCLE SYNCING

I RECENTLY TOOK A TRIP WITH MY HUSBAND AND PARENTS OUT TO California to visit my brother. While we were there, I caught up with friends old and new. When I met up with one friend, we started chatting about what I'd been up to. I shared the vision God put on my heart—to help women reclaim their identity in Christ and educate them on their menstrual cycles. She looked at me and said, "Kim, I've never told this to anyone, but for the past few years I haven't gotten my period. I feel so ashamed and long to feel like a woman again. I had no idea that I was overexercising and undereating and that I needed to switch up my diet to accommodate where I am in my cycle. Nobody ever told me this. What do I do?"

I've heard similar questions from many other women. Fortunately, there are lots of resources on the different needs of the four cycle phases—menstrual, follicular, ovulatory, and luteal.

The term *cycle syncing* was first coined by Alisa Vitti, a functional nutrition and women's hormone expert who came up with the Cycle Syncing Method. According to her website, cycle syncing is "the proprietary framework, founded by Alisa Vitta of FLO Living, that matches food, workouts and lifestyle with your cycle phases so that you can feel your best, every day of the month."[1] In this chapter we'll walk through each phase and explore best practices for living in hormonal harmony from a food and lifestyle perspective, all with Jesus at the center!

As you step into the world of cycle syncing, keep in mind that your body is wonderfully unique and may respond differently than that of the woman next to you. That's not just okay, that's by design. This is not a space for perfectionism or striving. Jesus doesn't call us to master a perfect routine; He calls us to *abide*. So let this journey be less about getting it "right" and more about noticing His fingerprints on your unique rhythms, trusting that even in the trial and error, He is gently shaping your steps.

Across the board, removing toxins from your life will dramatically improve your health. This may include changes to your cleaning and beauty products and a reduction or removal of synthetic clothing, processed foods, fragrances, plastics, and many other toxins we discussed previously. Changes in diet can be particularly hard, especially if you struggle with gut dysbiosis, which makes your tummy more sensitive to certain foods. It may be wise to partner with your practitioner to see which foods can work for you.

There is a ton of information to absorb, and if you're feeling a bit intimidated, you're not alone! Take things one step at a time. Doing it all at once can feel unsustainable and unenjoyable. This journey is meant to be inspiring, joyful, and grace-filled. So don't feel like you have to learn everything overnight; slow and steady wins the race.

THE MENSTRUAL PHASE

What's happening in your body:

- The corpus luteum gets reabsorbed by the body.
- The uterus sheds the endometrial lining, causing you to bleed.
- Hormones are at their lowest.

NUTRITION

Because your hormones are at their lowest when you're on your period, it's important to honor your body's cues for rest and repair. This is the winter phase, so warming, hearty foods are ideal, particularly ones rich in iron and magnesium. They're also comforting. Who wouldn't want a hot bowl of soup while curled up on the couch? Because of blood loss and lower energy levels, try to eat plenty of protein and healthy fats—they're essential for hormone production.

Some women report feeling colder during this phase, which makes sense considering the absence of estrogen (a naturally warming hormone). You may find cooked vegetables and slow-roasted foods satisfying and nourishing. It's normal to feel inflamed or "puffy" because of the uterine lining shedding, so adding anti-inflammatory foods might help calm the inflammation.

Consider adding some of these foods in this phase:

- Whole grains
- Soups/stews
- Flaxseed
- Pumpkin seeds
- Walnuts
- Dark, mixed greens
- Beets
- Kale
- Mushrooms
- Watermelon
- Wild rice
- Blackberries
- Blueberries
- Pork
- Lobster
- Scallops
- Red meat
- Kidney beans
- Bone broth
- Oily fish
- Dark chocolate

It pains me to say, but you might want to avoid coffee and fried, fatty foods. I know. I'm also rolling my eyes, because I crave a lot of fried foods when on my period. But both can work against your hormones, activating your body's stress response. Caffeine is a vasoconstrictor, meaning it narrows blood vessels, including those in the uterus, which can intensify cramps and increase discomfort during your bleed. Caffeine also spikes cortisol and can worsen PMS symptoms like breast tenderness and irritability.

Fried, fatty foods (especially those drenched in seed oils) are proinflammatory, acting as fuel to the already existing inflammation fire. They interfere with prostaglandins—the hormone-like substances responsible for cramping—and are high in omega-6s, which can throw off hormone balance. These foods can also make the liver more sluggish, leading to less than optimal estrogen detoxification, and sometimes cause a blood sugar roller coaster.

LIFESTYLE

When it comes to movement, take it easy. Lighter, restorative exercises often serve you best in this season, even if you feel capable of pushing harder. Listen to your body and honor what it's telling you. The key words here are low-impact, low-intensity, and low-stress. The last thing you want is a cortisol spike from exercise overload. Remember, Jesus often stepped away from the crowds to rest and be renewed in the Father's presence. If your period is a time for peace, then your workouts can mirror the same rhythm. Taking it down a notch isn't about losing progress or falling behind; it's about receiving the Lord's invitation in Matthew 11:28–30 to be yoked to Him, for His yoke is easy and His burden is light.

Here are some ways to move your body while on your period:

- Walking (solo, with a friend, or in prayer with Jesus)
- Pilates, especially core stability and pelvic floor support
- Stretching, focusing on hip openers and lower back relief

- Somatic breath work, inhaling for four counts, holding for seven, exhaling for eight
- Foam rolling or mobility work

Your menstrual phase serves as a reminder that rest isn't wasted time. In this slower season, your body is quietly doing the deep work of repair and your spirit has a chance to draw nearer to Jesus without the constant noise of "doing."

THE FOLLICULAR PHASE

What's happening in your body:

- FSH stimulates follicles in the ovaries to mature.
- Estrogen rises as it gets the uterus ready for a potential fertilized egg.
- LH releases to support the follicles to maturation.
- Energy levels rapidly climb.

NUTRITION

One of the best ways to support your body during the follicular phase is by loading up on antioxidant-rich, anti-inflammatory foods and incorporating plenty of pre- and probiotics. Your body has just spent days exerting energy on your period, and now it's ready to rebuild. Estrogen and gut health are closely linked, and as the "hype girl" rises in you, the gut microbiome—especially the estrobolome—plays a key role in breaking down and eliminating excess estrogen from the body. An unhealthy gut can cause estrogen to recirculate in unfavorable ways, resulting in bloating, mood swings, heavier periods, and estrogen dominance in the luteal phase. Probiotics are beneficial bacteria that support a healthy gut flora, which can reduce inflammation and indirectly aid in estrogen metabolism by giving the microbiome more support. Prebiotics act as the food that nourishes these good bacteria, helping them grow and thrive. And because 70 to 80 percent of your immune system is located in your gut, the foods you eat in this phase not only affect your hormones but also fortify your body's God-given defenses.[2]

When you nourish yourself this way, you're not just "eating healthy"—you're working with the Lord's design for healing, restoration, and flourishing. Each meal becomes a small act of worship, a way to say, "Thank You, Lord, for the body You've given me. Help me care for it well."

Try incorporating some of these foods during your next follicular phase:

Prebiotic Foods

- Onion
- Garlic
- Asparagus
- Chickpeas
- Lentils
- Apples
- Bananas
- Flaxseed
- Chia seeds

Probiotic Foods

- Yogurt
- Kefir
- Kimchi
- Sauerkraut
- Pickles
- Miso
- Tempeh
- Kombucha

Anti-Inflammatory Foods

- Turmeric
- Ginger
- Cilantro
- Berries, cherries, citrus, pomegranate
- Leafy greens (spinach, kale, arugula)
- Cruciferous veggies (broccoli, cauliflower)
- Sweet potato, squash, beets
- Bell peppers, red cabbage
- Fatty fish (salmon, sardines, mackerel)
- Chia seeds, flaxseed, walnuts
- Avocado, olive oil
- Oats, brown rice, quinoa, barley
- Herbal teas (nettle, chasteberry, raspberry leaf, chamomile, etc.)

LIFESTYLE

With a surge of estrogen comes a rise in energy, creativity, motivation, optimism, and exploration—God's way of giving your body the green light to move, create, and engage. This is the time to push yourself with workouts. You'll even recover faster! You may feel more social during this phase, so grab a friend and try a new class or activity together—community and movement is a win-win. The building of muscle is crucial for women's health, especially for those with PCOS or other metabolic issues. It improves blood sugar stability, helps regulate estrogen and progesterone, protects thyroid health, and makes you more resilient to stress, equipping you to walk out the purposes God has for you with strength and endurance. You don't have to go out and start lifting hundreds of pounds (please don't); starting with body weight is more than enough. Aim for two to three times a week, but listen to your body when it tells you to speed up or slow down.

Additional workout ideas:

- Go on a hike to a place with a view.
- Ride a bike along a pretty trail.
- Strength train with body weight or weights.
- Try a new workout class (barre, indoor cycling, Pilates, etc.).
- Go for a run.
- Swim laps.
- Dance.
- Try a new sport (pickleball, volleyball, tennis, etc.).

In every phase, whether your body is feeling strong, sluggish, or somewhere in between, remember that movement is a gift, not something to force yourself to do or punish yourself with. As you step into each workout, let it be less about chasing perfection and more about partnering with God in the stewardship of the vessel He's entrusted to you.

THE OVULATORY PHASE

What's happening in your body:

- LH rapidly surges and bursts open one mature follicle.

- The dominant egg starts the journey through the fallopian tubes to the uterus.
- The uterine lining becomes thicker.
- Estrogen reaches its peak.
- Testosterone surges, then goes back down.
- Your peak fertility window opens.

NUTRITION

As we learned in chapter 2, the ovulatory phase is the summer phase, a season of warmth, radiance, and connection—with others and with God. For nutrition, consider light, airy, hydrating, juicy, colorful foods you'd want to gobble down on a hot August day. Imagine you're sitting by the pool. What would you reach for? Maybe a smoothie bowl, a cold salad, or some juicy watermelon. The same rules apply here! Your liver is the unsung hero in this phase, helping to detoxify excess estrogen so your hormones stay balanced. God created bitter foods—like radicchio, arugula, watercress, and kale—not only to add flavor but to bless your liver's work.

These foods are especially nourishing for your body during ovulation:

- Brussels sprouts
- Eggplant
- Spinach
- Tomato
- Apricots
- Strawberries
- Raspberries
- Pomegranates
- Almonds
- Pecans
- Lamb
- Pasture-raised chicken or turkey
- Broccoli

- Bell peppers
- Cabbage
- Cauliflower
- Wild-caught salmon
- Eggs
- Avocado

LIFESTYLE

If the follicular phase was a ramp-up phase, ovulation is a time to go full throttle (within reason, of course). This is your peak window of energy, motivation, and endurance, so lean into it with gratitude. For some, that might mean reaching a new personal record in the gym; for others, it might be doing cardio that leaves you dripping in sweat and smiling from ear to ear. Whatever it is, choose movement that brings you joy. But even in celebrating your physical strength, recognize that it is the Lord who renews your spirit (Isaiah 40:31). Go all out, but keep your eyes on the One who gave you that strength in the first place.

Here are some ideas for your next ovulatory phase:

- Strength training (lifting heavier weights)
- High-intensity interval training (HIIT) (sprint intervals, circuit workouts, etc.)
- Cardio (stair-climbing, running, or sled-pushing)
- Group fitness classes (Zumba, salsa, etc.)
- Sports (pickup basketball, soccer, tennis, etc.)
- Cross-training

In the ovulatory phase, your body is firing on all cylinders thanks to estrogen and testosterone. Your hormones are essentially chanting, "Let's do this!" So lean into this moment and embrace challenging, joy-filled movements.

You may even be surprised at what your body is capable of. In this season, your workouts aren't just about building physical endurance; they're an opportunity to praise the Lord with your whole being, honoring Him with the way you honor your body.

THE LUTEAL PHASE

What's happening in your body:

- → The corpus luteum produces progesterone.
- → Estrogen slightly dips, then rises in the middle of the phase before dipping back down.
- → Your body determines whether pregnancy has occurred.
- → PMS symptoms arise if estrogen is too high and progesterone is too low.

NUTRITION

Whether or not you're pregnant, your body was designed to rely on healthy progesterone production in this phase. Many women silently battle estrogen dominance, which can bring on all those frustrating PMS symptoms we know too well. During these two weeks, your body is more sensitive to changes in blood sugar, so it's wise to incorporate more low-glycemic, whole foods to help keep levels steady without sending your body into a roller coaster of spikes and crashes. Complex carbohydrates, like sweet potatoes, butternut squash, pumpkin, beets, brown rice, millet, buckwheat, amaranth, farro, oats, and wild rice, slow the release of glucose, supporting both insulin and hormone balance.

And then there's fiber—a nutrient God's creation is overflowing with, yet most of us are barely getting 5 percent of what we need daily (about twenty-five grams).[3] Fiber is a humble but powerful servant: It sweeps out excess hormones, keeps digestion moving, feeds the gut, supports healthy weight, and helps maintain steady blood sugar. In short, it's one of the simplest God-given tools for whole-body health. We need more fiber!

Health tip: Pair fiber with healthy fats and protein to keep sugar cravings at bay!

Here's a list of fiber-rich foods to incorporate during your luteal phase:

- → Carrots
- → Broccoli
- → Brussels sprouts
- → Kale
- → Cauliflower
- → Blueberries
- → Raspberries
- → Strawberries
- → Apples
- → Pears
- → Figs
- → Oranges
- → Lentils
- → Chickpeas
- → Black beans
- → Pumpkin seeds
- → Chia seeds
- → Flaxseed

LIFESTYLE

While the ovulatory phase invites you to go full throttle, the luteal phase calls you into slower, more intentional rhythms. Progesterone rises, your body shifts toward restoration, and your energy becomes more grounded. Lean into gentler, more grounding forms of movement that support your nervous system and keep stress low. Think strengthening, stabilizing, and lower-intensity workouts that make you feel supported rather than spent. Prioritize sleep, incorporate more quiet time, and build margins into your days instead of packing them to overflow. This phase is where you naturally turn more inward, making it a beautiful time to connect with your body and the Lord in an intentional way.

Here are some ideas for your next luteal phase:

- Pilates (reformer or mat)
- Strength training (Use just body weight or lighter weights and higher reps)
- Stretching
- Deep-breathing exercises
- Long walks

In this phase, think of movement as grounding rather than pushing. You're honoring your body's cues to slow down, giving it what it needs instead of forcing what it doesn't. As you get ready to move your body, take a deep breath and remember that it's often in the stillness that God's presence is felt most.

SUPPLEMENTS AND KEY NUTRIENTS THROUGHOUT YOUR CYCLE

Before we step into the wild, wild world of supplements, let's start with a gentle reminder: Your body is unique, and what works wonders for one person may not be the right fit for you. That's why it's wise to have a full nutrient blood panel done before starting anything new. This gives you (and your provider) a clear picture of where your levels are and what your body truly needs. Supplements can be a powerful tool in pulling your body out of a deficiency, but taking too much or taking the wrong type can be harmful. It's also important to note that some supplements aren't as effective as others, so it's worth doing your research, reading labels carefully, seeking medical supervision from a trusted doctor or nutritionist, and choosing high-quality, third party–tested brands that your body can absorb and use effectively. This way, you're not simply downing pills—you're truly nourishing your body.

One of the most common questions I hear from my online community and clients is, "What supplements should I take to fix my hormones?" My honest answer is always, "It depends." In my training as a certified integrative nutritionist and hormone health coach, I've learned that our health is rarely one-dimensional. Symptoms are often the surface ripples of deeper imbalances—nutritional, hormonal, emotional, or even spiritual. That's why I appreciate that integrative medicine looks at the whole person, not only the lab results, and offers both holistic and medicinal solutions.

While supplementation will look different for each person, several vitamins tend to yield positive results for me and the clients I've worked with: vitamin C, vitamin D, omega-3 fatty acid, and magnesium glycinate. Each plays a vital role in hormone production and regulation, and deficiencies in these are more common than most of us realize.

While this isn't a one-size-fits-all prescription, it's a starting point we can explore together—always with wisdom from the Holy Spirit, prayer, and a willingness to listen to what your body is telling you.

VITAMIN C

Vitamin C (ascorbic acid) is a water-soluble vitamin essential for immune function, collagen production, hormone health, adrenal support, detoxification, and antioxidant support. Because the body can't make this vitamin on its own, it must come from food or supplementation. As a powerful antioxidant, vitamin C helps neutralize free radicals, protecting cells from oxidative stress, calming inflammation, and supporting tissue repair. It's also essential for collagen synthesis, which keeps skin, joints, and bones healthy. The highest concentrations of vitamin C are found in the adrenal glands, reflecting its important role in stress response. Has anyone offered you a vitamin C pack from the drugstore when you're feeling sick? That's because vitamin C supports immune health by reducing histamine production for allergy relief and enhancing the production of white blood cells. Your immune system is one of God's incredible gifts—a built-in defense team He designed to fight for you daily, whether or not you notice it. Just as God promises to go before you and fight your battles in the world (Deuteronomy 20:4), He is also faithfully waging those battles within you, protecting and sustaining you in ways you can't always see.

The following is a list of possible signs of a vitamin C deficiency:

- Frequent infections
- Poor wound healing
- Easy bruising
- Bleeding gums
- Rough, dry skin
- Joint pain or stiffness
- Low progesterone symptoms
- Fatigue or low energy

If supplementation is not your thing and you'd rather try adding more vitamin C to your diet instead, consider filling your plate with some of the following:

- Kiwi
- Strawberries
- Oranges
- Red and yellow bell peppers
- Broccoli
- Brussels sprouts
- Kale
- Acerola cherries (extremely high in vitamin C)

VITAMIN D

Nearly two thirds of American adults have insufficient vitamin D levels.[4] Vitamin D is a powerhouse for health, aiding in bone support, immune function, hormone production and regulation, gene expression, and cardiovascular health. More than just a nutrient, vitamin D is classified as a secosteroid, meaning it functions much like a hormone in the body, influencing systems far beyond bone health. And here's the awe-inspiring part: God designed our skin with the ability to produce this vital compound when sunlight touches it. He made the sun to sustain life on earth, and that same sun plays a role in sustaining hormonal health. Receptors for this vitamin are found in the ovaries, pituitary gland, uterus, and hypothalamus—parts of the body that work together to keep our cycles in balance. Without enough vitamin D, this beautiful communication system can weaken, which may lead to menstrual struggles. And just as sunlight nourishes the earth, vitamin D helps our bodies absorb calcium, keeping our bones strong and our bodies steady.[5]

If you suspect you may be deficient in vitamin D, look for these signs:

→ Fatigue
→ Frequent illness
→ Menstrual irregularities
→ PCOS
→ Fertility challenges
→ Depression or low mood
→ Bone pain
→ Muscle aches
→ Hair loss
→ Poor blood sugar regulation

The best way to get more vitamin D is by increasing your time in the sun (while taking precautions against sunburn). Some animal-based foods like cod-liver oil, beef liver, wild-caught salmon, tuna, and Swiss cheese contain vitamin D3, the most bioavailable and effective form of vitamin D. Though debated in the medical field for its efficacy, vitamin D supplementation may move the needle for some. That's why it's wise to combine it with time in the sun and vitamin D–rich foods to ensure you're getting all your body needs to thrive.

OMEGA-3 FATTY ACID

Are you aware that when you're pregnant, the fat stored in your butt, hips, and thighs is what contributes to the development of your baby's brain? Yes, you read that right! The areas of our body we spend years picking apart, pinching in disgust, and wishing away are full of healthy omega-3 fats that aid in the building of your baby's brain. What's even cooler is that those fat tissues are preserved until you're in late pregnancy and while breastfeeding postpartum, because your body intentionally holds on to those DHA-rich stores so it can keep fueling your baby's brain long after birth. So think about that the next time you want to talk negatively about your body!

Omega-3s are essential fats, meaning your body can't make them on its own and they must come from diet or supplements. There are three types: ALA, EPA, and DHA, with the last two being the most bioavailable and used most effectively in the body. Omega-3 fatty acid reduces inflammation, making it a great fit for those with PCOS, endometriosis, painful periods, insulin resistance, or autoimmune conditions. It plays a key role in supporting brain health and stabilizing mood, with evidence showing it can help ease PMS symptoms.[6] It enhances hormone balance by improving communication within the endocrine system, reducing unhealthy fats (triglycerides), boosting insulin sensitivity, and supporting fertility and healthy pregnancies. DHA is vital for egg quality, embryo growth, and the development of a baby's eyes and brain.[7]

Omega-3s play a crucial role, but their balance with omega-6s is just as important. Your body needs both, but often our Western diets include an excessive amount of omega-6.[8] An optimal ratio is 4:1 (omega-6: omega-3), but in America we see ratios upward of 25:1. Think of omega-6s as the fire starter (inflammatory) and omega-3s as the water that keeps the fire in check (anti-inflammatory). Seed oils—like vegetable, canola, corn, safflower, soybean—are high in omega-6s and can be one of the main contributors to inflammation in the body. When the ratio of omega-6s to omega-3s is too high, you may experience painful periods, cramping, skin issues, worsened symptoms of PCOS, endometriosis, or chronic inflammation. That's because omega-6s prompt your body to create prostaglandins.

There are three prostaglandins: PGE1, PGE2, and PGE3. If you experience intense cramping, it's because of PGE2. It is produced as an inflammatory response. But get this: PGE1 and PGE3 are the antidote to cramps. God gives us a *double portion* for healing period cramps! Can I get an amen?

These symptoms may be signs of low omega-3 fatty acid:

- Irregular, painful periods
- Severe cramping

- Fertility struggles
- Chronic inflammation
- Excessive hair shedding
- Dry, flaky skin
- Anxiety or irritability
- Mood swings (especially around the luteal phase)
- High triglycerides
- Insulin resistance
- Fatigue after meals
- Dry eyes

If you're looking for a more natural route to add omega-3s, try these foods:

- Cod-liver oil
- Wild-caught salmon
- Sardines
- Anchovies
- Chia seeds
- Ground flaxseed
- Walnuts
- Hemp seeds
- Brussels sprouts

To give your body the best shot at improving your omega-6 to omega-3 ratio, first eliminate highly processed foods that have undergone chemical processing, bleaching, or deodorizing, and sustained high levels of heating. While shopping at the grocery store, before tossing any chip or snack bag in the cart, flip the packaging around to its ingredient label to check what the first three ingredients are. If it's a vegetable oil–based product, consider swapping to one that uses avocado oil or olive oil. A general rule of thumb is that if you can't pronounce the ingredient, it was likely added in the processing stage. You don't need to eliminate seed oils completely—in fact, it's highly contested among professionals—but they should be consumed in moderation.

MAGNESIUM GLYCINATE

Magnesium is finally getting the recognition it deserves. It is involved in over three hundred enzymatic reactions in the body, including producing hormones, managing stress, improving sleep, and boosting metabolism. "In fact, a 2018 study published in *The Journal of the American Osteopathic Association* suggests that up to 50 percent of the U.S. population may be magnesium-deficient."[9] According to the National Institutes of Health, "Low levels of magnesium have been associated with a number of chronic diseases, such as Alzheimer's disease, insulin resistance and type-2 diabetes mellitus, hypertension, cardiovascular disease (e.g., stroke), migraine headaches, and attention deficit hyperactivity disorder (ADHD)."[10] Magnesium glycinate is a specific form bound to glycine, an amino acid with calming, antianxiety effects. It also has an impact on reproductive health, due to its calming effects on the brain and muscles, and it can be incredibly helpful for easing cramps and period discomfort. Philippians 4:7 promises a peace that will "guard your hearts and your minds in Christ Jesus," and magnesium can be one of the physical tools God has given us to experience more calmness and stability in our daily lives.

Other hormone-supporting benefits include boosting progesterone production, easing symptoms linked to low progesterone—such as anxiety, spotting, and poor sleep—helping regulate the HPA axis by lowering cortisol levels, and enhancing insulin sensitivity. For my PMDD, magnesium glycinate was the first supplement that moved the needle for symptom relief.

Look out for these signs if you sense you might be low in magnesium:

- "On edge" feeling
- Anxiety
- Insomnia or restless sleep
- Low progesterone–related PMS symptoms
- Headaches
- Sugar cravings and imbalanced blood sugar
- Period cramps

Outside of supplements, the following foods contain high levels of magnesium. Consider adding them to your plate this week:

- Dark leafy greens
- Watermelon
- Pumpkin seeds
- Black beans
- Edamame
- Almonds
- Butternut squash

God has truly given us everything we need within us and in His creation to heal and thrive. He also uses medical professionals, naturopathic doctors, functional practitioners, health coaches, and many other healers to come alongside us on our health journey, offering wisdom and answers to problems we may have felt trapped in. The body is extraordinarily complex, and your health issues might not be fixable or even improvable through diet, lifestyle, or supplements alone. That's not a reason *not* to try them, but keep in mind that healing is often a layered process. Sometimes healing requires medical intervention, and praise God that's an option. There's no right or wrong way to pursue health and wholeness; what matters is that you're faithfully following the path the Lord is leading you on.

Let's be women who tune in to our bodies, care for them, and nurture them by giving them the nutrients they need, all while learning to go with the flow (are you tired of these puns yet?). Extending yourself grace by knowing where you are in your cycle releases the pressure to push through and allows you to walk at a pace of peace, regardless of which phase you're in. Honoring your God-given body instead of battling it makes healing less about fixing and more about restoring. Your period isn't a curse; it's a compass guiding you toward health and wholeness. And you don't have to figure it all out at once. Just keep showing up with curiosity and an open heart, and the Lord will do the rest.

PRACTICAL APPLICATION

- → Try incorporating phase-specific foods into your diet to support your body throughout each stage of your cycle.
- → Consider getting a blood test to check for nutrient deficiencies.
- → Practice looking in the mirror and declaring God's truth over the areas of your body you struggle to love.

SCRIPTURE TO MEDITATE ON

→ "Those who hope in the Lord will renew their strength. They will soar on wings like eagles; they will run and not grow weary, they will walk and not be faint." (Isaiah 40:31)

TEN

STORE YOUR OIL

I LAY ON THE FLOOR OF MY BEDROOM AT MY PARENTS' HOUSE, frustrated and in tears over the season I was in. I was twenty-five years old with no job, which left me no choice but to move back in with my parents to save money. I went from a beautiful (but tiny) apartment in Manhattan back to my hometown in the suburbs of New Jersey.

This wasn't my plan. Moving home meant leaving behind all my friends, my church community, my favorite places to go for long walks, my go-to dinner spots, and the life I'd worked so hard to create. I found myself in an in-between season. One season had ended, and I had eight months until the next would begin. In the meantime, I had to move home.

Moving home felt like failure. It meant returning to a town that holds a lot of painful memories and living under my parents' rules as a full-grown adult with my own preferences and habits.

Of the numerous things I was afraid of, what my relationship with Jesus would look like worried me most. As a routine-oriented person, I had a great flow going with my God time. Each morning I'd wake up, make my bed, turn on worship music, brush my teeth, make breakfast, cozy up on the couch with my Bible, and journal for twenty minutes, then top it off with a thirty-minute prayer walk on the West Side Highway. This routine is what kept me grounded and rooted in the Word before the craziness of my work schedule began. I found solace in the predictability since my days were filled with chaos. Seeing the same joggers and passing the same buildings brought me comfort.

After my first few days of being home (and out of this routine), I was filled with anxiety. Where would I go for my morning walks? Where was the cozy corner in which I could read my Bible? What church would I attend? And where did my favorite mug go? Everything was different, from the scenery to the noises outside. Instead of ambulance sirens, I now heard birds chirping. Skyscrapers had been replaced with copy-and-paste houses with driveways and fancy landscaping.

Through the transition from Manhattan to the suburbs, God was teaching me an important lesson: Learn to go with the flow.

So there I was, knees digging into the carpet, head in hands as my tears spilled over.

"God, this is too much. I can't do this. How am I going to get through these next eight months?"

In a gentle whisper I heard the Holy Spirit say, "Store your oil."

I immediately knew that storing my oil meant being more intentional with my God time—reading Scripture more, spending even more time in prayer, remaining obedient even when I didn't necessarily want to, pausing more throughout the day to fix my eyes on Him—because there would be challenging moments when I'd need to tap into my "oil reserves" to keep me grounded. It was a beautiful acknowledgment that God knew this season would be hard for me yet a reminder that He was right there with me, leading me through each day.

I was so stuck in my routines that I wasn't leaving room for God to work in me. A big part of why I was so adamant about my morning routine was that I felt like if I didn't spend time with Him first thing in the morning, then I had failed as a Christian. If I didn't listen to worship music right when I woke up, then I wouldn't be suited up with the armor of God. And if I didn't read the Word, then God would be upset with me. For so long I believed that spending time in His presence looked only one of four ways: worshipping through music, attending a Sunday service, praying, or reading the Bible.

This limited thinking has obvious issues because, one, God is not limited by *anything*. And two, on days when I simply didn't have the motivation to open the Bible or when I was crawling into Sunday service sick from exhaustion, I'd be crippled with guilt.

"I should want to read my Bible."

"I should have the motivation to war in prayer."

"What's wrong with me?"

"Am I a bad Christian?"

And then it hit me: I was going against my very design by forcing myself to make something work when my body simply couldn't handle it. Just as I needed to lean into the season of living at my parents' house, I needed to lean into my hormonal seasons too.

In chapter 9 we learned about cycle syncing—using food and lifestyle to our advantage based on each phase of our cycle. Now we're going to zoom in on the spiritual component so we can go with our flow to optimize our motivation, preserve our energy, and savor the sweet moments of rest to move out of a place of guilt-driven worship and into purehearted praise each day of the month. And we're going to learn how to store our oil so we feel spiritually covered and prepared before each new phase begins—because for everything there is a season.

THE MENSTRUAL PHASE: A TIME FOR PEACE

The key word for the menstrual phase is *rest*. Your body's inability to keep up with your normal speed is an indicator that it's time to slow down. I've learned the hard way (one too many times) that pushing myself past what I can handle only leads to more frustration and anger. And I'd argue that it leaves me feeling worse than before. If you've ever tried to go for a run on your period and noticed that you're more out of breath than usual, there's a reason for it. All signals are blinking red, and Jesus is inviting you to enter His place of rest.

Let's do a little exercise together: Close your eyes and imagine you're on day 2 of your period. Take notice of any sensations, feelings, pain, or discomfort you feel. Check in with your energy levels: Are you feeling fired up, tired, sleepy, excited? Assess your mental state: Are you stressed, anxious, worried, irritable, happy, hopeful?

To help a friend feel better in this situation, what would you recommend she do? Maybe you'd suggest a movie night, offer a shoulder to cry on, or encourage her to journal, read a book, or eat a bowl of hearty soup? You would probably tell her to rest.

What if Jesus is telling you the same thing?

Our relationship with Jesus doesn't have to look different than our relationship with our friends. It can really be that simple. If the thought of attending a high-energy worship night feels overwhelming, stay home and listen to worship music while you journal. Or if the idea of sharing in your small group is too much to handle, watch a sermon on YouTube instead. We can easily get caught up in guilt over feeling like we're not *doing enough* for God. But He never asks us to have a lengthy checklist of Christian activities that we must check off daily. His desire is for us to spend quality time with Him.

I love the story of Mary and Martha of Bethany so much that I have to bring them up again. Upon Jesus's arrival at their home, Martha immediately began cleaning the house, cooking the meal, and preparing the table, while Mary "sat at the Lord's feet listening to what he said" (Luke 10:39). Martha said to Jesus, "Lord, don't you care that my sister has left me to do the work by myself? Tell her to help me!"

(v. 40). Jesus answered, "Martha . . . you are worried and upset about many things, but few things are needed—or indeed only one. Mary has chosen what is better, and it will not be taken away from her" (vv. 41–42).

Notice that Martha was *doing* while Mary was *sitting* at Jesus's feet. Mary rested in the presence of God. Our periods are reminders that there's a time to push, but now is the time to prioritize rest and recovery.

The truth is that we could never do enough to fully repay Jesus for His sacrifice. If we're stuck in a mindset of constantly working and doing to please God, we're missing the whole point of why Jesus came in the first place. He came so we could have a relationship with Him. And all He wants is our hearts and minds fully set on Him.

Jesus loves quality time, so what better opportunity to set aside our striving than when we're on our period? Here are a few ideas for getting in His presence while in your menstrual phase:

- → Cozy up on the couch and read the Word.
- → Sit in silence.
- → Journal with a candle lit.
- → Play worship music while you go about your daily tasks.
- → Cook a homemade meal and have dinner with Jesus.
- → Watch a sermon on YouTube.
- → FaceTime a friend for a mini Bible study.
- → Sabbath—Put your phone down for one day a week to focus on being present.

I want to remind you that resting doesn't equal weakness. The Bible mentions the word *rest* hundreds of times. And if Jesus needed to step away from daily activities to spend time with His Father, how much more do we? As a society we've normalized hustle culture, and this mindset bleeds into our relationship with God. Our good works should always come from the overflow of our intimacy with Jesus. We don't need to do more, like Martha; we need to sit at Jesus's feet, like Mary.

THE FOLLICULAR PHASE: A TIME TO DANCE

The follicular phase is the time to take advantage of your feel-good energy and sociability. Even though three days ago you may have wanted to shout at your neighbor, today you may feel like you want to serve them by offering to go grocery shopping for them. Remember, this is a season of bloom. Use this time to think big, get creative, and mark up your spiritual drawing board.

One of my favorite things to do to feel close to God during the follicular phase is spending time in nature. This looks like going on long walks, hikes, or bike rides or simply lying in the backyard watching the sunset. Psalm 19:1 says, "The heavens declare the glory of God; the skies proclaim the work of his hands."

Just as we reflect the image of God (the *imago Dei*), creation reflects His creativity and splendor. Each time I see sunrays beaming down through the cracks of a cloudy sky,

I well up with tears. I imagine Jesus's arms stretched wide from heaven, offering me a warm embrace.

When God seems silent, step outside. Smell the fresh air. Look at the beautiful trees blowing and bending gently in the wind. Feel the sun's rays dancing on your face. Listen to the birds singing and chirping. Take your shoes off and walk barefoot in the grass, feeling each blade tickle the bottoms of your feet. Sink your hands into the sand, taking notice of how tiny each grain truly is.

> How precious to me are your thoughts, God!
> How vast is the sum of them!
> Were I to count them,
> they would outnumber the grains of sand—
> when I awake, I am still with you.
> (Psalm 139:17–18)

Leave room for the Holy Spirit to bring Scripture to your mind or speak revelation to you. God is everywhere, but sometimes we forget how easy He is to find.

It's no coincidence that nature is healing for our bodies. Each time you sit next to a waterfall, walk barefoot in the grass, or sit on the beach looking out at the waves, you soak up negative ions. These grounding techniques have been shown to reduce inflammation, reduce cortisol, improve sleep and circadian rhythm, and improve blood flow.[1]

Try incorporating one of these spiritual practices the next time you're in the follicular phase:

- → Join a community group at church.
- → Set new personal and spiritual goals.
- → Start a new Bible reading plan.
- → Volunteer to serve on a team.
- → Tap into your creative giftings.
- → Go for a prayer walk in your local park or neighborhood.
- → Take a hike to a place with a view.
- → Sit on the beach and listen to the sound of the ocean.
- → Lie in your backyard and stargaze.

Worship can happen anywhere at any time because God is omnipresent and His Spirit lives inside us. Things like connecting with nature and tapping into our creative giftings (singing, painting, dancing, etc.) allow us to experience God's design on a deeper, more intimate level.

THE OVULATORY PHASE: A TIME TO EMBRACE

The ovulatory phase is the best time to embrace the abundance of joy, love, and grace and to sow it back into the kingdom. Praying bold prayers, engaging in intercession, worshipping out loud, and getting in groups are great ways to take advantage of your fruitful hormonal profile. All these things add to your stored oil so that when you downshift into the luteal phase, you have reserves to tap into.

I want to challenge you to love others radically. Get in the secret place with God and ask Him to reveal things that have been hidden to you: people you need to forgive, let go of, or move on from; lingering hurt that you need to release. Maybe you need to schedule a tough conversation with someone you love. Putting yourself out there can be scary, but you can do anything through Christ who strengthens you.

During your next ovulatory phase, I encourage you to try one of these spiritual practices:

- → Pray bold prayers.
- → Engage in intercession.
- → Connect with your spouse (date night).
- → Forgive where forgiveness is due.
- → Volunteer to serve at your church's next event.
- → Attend a worship night.
- → Pay for a stranger's coffee.
- → Call a friend or family member and tell them you love them.
- → Display a random act of kindness.
- → Ask to sit with the person who always sits alone.

Connecting with others is a direct way to connect with God Himself. Jesus demonstrated this through His life, coming not to be served but to serve (Matthew 20:28). All throughout Scripture we see God's servanthood on display. And one way to serve is through acts of love and service. Genesis to Revelation is God's love note to us. Now it's your turn to write a love note to others.

THE LUTEAL PHASE: A TIME TO PLANT

As your body downshifts in the luteal phase, turn your focus from outward to inward. This is the perfect time to ask the Lord to check your heart. Pray David's prayer in Psalm 139:

> Search me, God, and know my heart;
> test me and know my anxious thoughts.
> See if there is any offensive way in me,
> and lead me in the way everlasting. (vv. 23–24)

Consider the luteal phase a season of pruning.

My favorite way to spend time with Jesus in the luteal phase is to journal. I often find that after I've written down all my thoughts, fears, and emotions, God takes the pen and begins writing a message to me. In that in-between season I described, it looked a little like this:

"Lord, I'm feeling anxious about living at home. I don't want to be here; I'm getting triggered repeatedly by the memories in this house, and I feel like I'm a teenager again. I miss my independence and having my own space."

And God would begin to move in my heart:

My daughter, I see how hard it is for you to be here. But I am right here with you. I want you to have a different perspective on being home, and I want to heal the broken parts of you that are lodged in your heart. I have not forsaken you, nor will I ever abandon you. Please trust that I have a plan for this season and know that I love you so much.

God wants to dialogue with us. He tore the veil of the temple once and for all so we can have 24/7 access to Him. And He wants us to know Him and put our trust in Him. Don't be afraid to go to Him with your doubt or anger. There's nothing you could ever say to Him that would surprise Him.

We'll each have many bad days, but we can have them in front of God. He wants to be invited into every area of our lives. Not only the bright and shiny, but the ugly and gritty too. If you never open up to a friend about a struggle you're facing, how will she know how to comfort you? If you never tell your spouse when they've hurt your feelings, how will you ever reconcile and move forward? If you never share the thoughts and feelings you want to tuck away and keep hidden from God, how will you ever experience His supernatural and indescribable love and peace? He is a good Father who desires good things for His children. We must be willing to slow down, look inward, and then look upward.

Consider adding one of these spiritual practices to your routine the next time your luteal phase rolls around:

- Shift from *doing* to *being*.
- Journal about your emotions and frustrations.
- Write a letter from God to you.
- Spend time in silence and solitude.
- Read the Word with a warm cup of coffee or tea.
- Pray for revelation.
- Talk openly to Jesus about how you truly feel.
- Pray David's prayer in Psalm 139.
- Lean on a friend for support and encouragement.

The Lord collects our tears in a bottle (Psalm 56:8 NLT). We have a loving Father who sees every tear, hears every cry, and comforts all those who are brokenhearted. Let this be a time to trust-fall into the arms of your heavenly Father. Allow Him the space to comfort, guide, and lead you to His still waters.

You may have been taught to believe that worship exists only when you're happy, "feeling" like you want to, or is found in the four walls of a church, but worship can happen anywhere, under any circumstances, and at any time because the Spirit lives inside you. This means that wherever you go and whoever you interact with, you can worship the Lord through your words and actions, regardless of where you are in your cycle. Even when you're moody, tired, or impatient, God can use you. For every season—resting, dancing, embracing, planting—He's present. Even when you feel out of sync, His Spirit within you keeps the rhythm. Nothing in your cycle, your emotions, or your body disqualifies you from worship; instead, these become offerings that draw you nearer to the One who holds all seasons in His hands.

And this is what it means to store your oil: worshipping in the ordinary, surrendering even the small moments, and letting God fill your lamp, drop by drop. When the time comes, the oil you've stored—through obedience, prayer, rest, and faithfulness—will keep your light burning bright. Your body may change, your seasons may shift, but when you choose worship through all of it, you're not only sustaining yourself but also preparing for the Bridegroom with oil in your lamp and a heart that is ready (Matthew 25:1–13).

PRACTICAL APPLICATION

- Choose a new spiritual practice from each phase and incorporate them throughout the next four phases of your cycle.
- Pick up a pen and journal your anxious thoughts.
- Write a love letter to yourself from God.
- Invite community into your life for encouragement, support, and accountability.
- Memorize one verse of Scripture from this chapter and meditate on it throughout the week.

SCRIPTURE TO MEDITATE ON

- "How precious to me are your thoughts, God! How vast is the sum of them! Were I to count them, they would outnumber the grains of sand—when I awake, I am still with you." (Psalm 139:17–18)
- "Search me, God, and know my heart; test me and know my anxious thoughts. See if there is any offensive way in me, and lead me in the way everlasting." (Psalm 139:23–24)
- "The heavens declare the glory of God; the skies proclaim the work of his hands." (Psalm 19:1)

ELEVEN

SLOW IS STILL HOLY

I USED TO BELIEVE THAT REST WAS A REWARD, SOMETHING deserved after a long day's work. But then I'd find myself drowning in to-do lists. And even though my hours were filled to the brim, I guilted myself for not doing more. So I didn't rest.

Failure.

No reward.

No rest.

The cycle would continue and eventually look something like this:

Drown in responsibilities.

Complete to-do list.

Rest.

Guilt self for not getting started on the *other* list.

Get up off the couch and push through.

Guilt self for not resting.

Day after day this mental tug-of-war wore on more than just my body—it eroded my sense of worth. My identity was entangled in productivity, and rest wasn't refreshing anymore. It was a mental war zone. If I sat down, I felt lazy. If I got up, I felt exhausted. If I paused, I felt like I was falling behind. And then came the racing thoughts at night, the jolt of panic.

During this struggle, I came across an Instagram post that deeply moved me. It read, "Growing up, I never knew a relaxed woman. Successful women? Yes. Productive women? Plenty. Anxious and afraid and apologetic women? Heaps of them. But relaxed women? At-ease women? Women who don't dissect their days into half-hour slots of productivity? Women who prioritize rest and pleasure and play? Women who aren't afraid to take up space in the world? Women who give themselves unconditional permission to relax? Without guilt? Without apology? Without feeling like they need to earn it? I'm not sure I've ever met a woman like that. But I would like to become one."[1]

This quote from Nicola Jane Hobbs punched me in the gut. Surely I could think of at least one woman in my life who knew how to relax and take time for herself. But I found I couldn't name one. I realized that this wasn't just a *me* problem, it was a *we* problem.

The American Psychological Association performed a study in 2023 on three thousand adults, and the results are shocking (but not surprising):

→ Women reported a higher average level of stress than men (5.3 out of 10 compared with men's 4.8).

- → Women were more likely to report their stress levels between 8 and 10.
- → Women were more likely to say they "strongly agree" that no one understands how stressed they are.
- → Women reported that they do not get over stress quickly.
- → Women noted family responsibilities and relationships as key stressors in their lives (58 percent of women versus 52 percent of men).[2]

We're tired. We're mentally, physically, spiritually, and hormonally depleted. We often wear our exhaustion like a badge of honor and trick ourselves into believing rest is weakness. Many of our calendars are full, but our cups are empty. Yet we keep pushing, keep striving, and keep checking boxes, in part because we believe the only way to prove our worth is to earn it. But we don't need another productivity hack; we need a renewing of the mind.

What would it look like to reframe the way you see rest? What if you believed that it's something to freely receive? What if you allowed yourself to shift from striving and settle into stillness? What if we became women who didn't push through the period pain, the intense cramps, and the menstrual migraines? What would it look like if we listened to our bodies' cries for help?

You are worthy of rest because God made you worthy. You're not a machine, you're a daughter. Rest was never a fallback plan for burnout; it's God's blueprint for wholeness. He wove sabbath into creation before sin ever entered the world and called it *holy* (Genesis 2:2–3). He never asks you to earn it; He designed it because He knows how desperately you need it, especially in the context of your unique embodiment. And to truly understand this, you must go back to the garden.

WHEN GOD MADE EVE

Genesis reveals the story of creation and God's intentional design for every living thing on the earth, including the creation of human beings. The Lord made Adam from dust and placed him in the garden of Eden to tend and watch over the animals. But something was missing. Chapter 2 verse 18 tells us that God said, "It is not good for the man to be alone. I will make a helper suitable for him." So while Adam was sleeping, He took a piece of his rib and created woman. Eve was born. Her primary role was to be Adam's helper. The Hebrew word for "helper" is *ezer*, which, contrary to popular belief, does not mean servant, subordinate, or submissive sidekick. *Ezer* is a divine word used twenty-one times in the Old Testament and is often used as a descriptor of Yahweh—our God. One of the times it is used in that context is in Deuteronomy 33:26, 29 (NLT) in Moses's song to the Hebrew people before he died:

> There is no one like the God of Israel.
> He rides across the heavens to help [*ezer*] you,
> across the skies in majestic splendor. . . .
> How blessed you are, O Israel!
> Who else is like you, a people saved by the Lord?

> He is your protecting shield [*ezer*]
> and your triumphant sword!
> Your enemies will cringe before you,
> and you will stomp on their backs!

Ezer is used here to describe God as a rescuer and protector. The imagery of a shield is also used in Psalms 33:20 and 115:9–11. Moses even named one of his sons Eliezer, meaning "My God is helper," and goes on to show God as the helper who delivered him from the sword of Pharaoh in Exodus 18:4. God even calls Himself *ezer* in Hosea 13:9: "You are destroyed, Israel, because you are against me, against your helper [*ezer*]."

Clearly God was not a docile assistant or submissive sidekick here!

God has given us a divine calling as *ezers*. We are a precious gift, sharing the likeness and character of Him who created us. And we weren't meant to exist in the shadow of a man; rather, we were created to come alongside, lift up, encourage, nurture, oversee, tend to, and care for others. This looks different for each woman, but the principle is the same: Be an ally, a helper for those in need. For some women this may mean raising children, tending to the home, or being a wife. For others this may look like leading with humility in the workplace, using skills and talents to glorify God, serving in community, mentoring younger women, leading small groups, donating time and resources to those in need, or volunteering in underserved neighborhoods. Each person plays an important role in the body of Christ.

One of Eve's roles was to comanage and oversee the animals, plants, and well-being of the planet. She was also Adam's divine partner, companion, equal. And considering God's design of marriage, she likely acted as a mirror to help Adam see his flaws and encourage him to grow more into holiness.

The Bible describes these additional traits of an *ezer*:

- → Of noble character (Proverbs 31:10–12)
- → Nurturing (Titus 2:4)
- → Faithful with resources (Proverbs 31:16–18)
- → Compassionate (Proverbs 31:19–22)
- → God-fearing (Proverbs 31:30)

The through line of biblical femininity is a heart that loves and serves God and His people. Christianity is perhaps the greatest feminist liberation of all time. When Jesus was here on earth, women were not seen as equals. Their voices were silenced, their witness wasn't legally recognized, and they were essentially confined by the authority of their husbands. Rabbinic oral law was clear: "He who talks with a woman [in public] brings evil upon himself."[3] Another prominent teaching of Jesus's day stated that one was not so much as to greet a woman.

So here came Jesus, talking and spending time with women in public. No wonder the disciples and religious leaders were stunned. Sue Bohlin of Probe Ministries goes on to say in her article titled "Christianity: The Best Thing to Ever Happen to Women" that the way Jesus responded to the Samaritan woman in John 4 may not seem radical to us, but He went directly against the cultural views that saw women as inferior. Even the Samaritan woman was shocked at His acknowledgment of her! Not only did Jesus speak to her, but He revealed Himself as the Messiah: "The woman said, 'I know that Messiah' (called Christ) 'is coming. When he comes, he will explain everything to us.' Then Jesus declared, 'I, the one speaking to you—I am he'" (John 4:25–26).

Sue continues her claim that Christianity is pro-female with the story of Mary, Martha, and Lazarus. When Lazarus died, Jesus comforted Martha and spoke the heart of the gospel to her—that He is the Way, the Truth, and the Life and whoever believes in that message will live forever. And then He asked her if she believed—an unspeakable act not only to teach a woman but to call for a verbal response. Once again Jesus flipped the way the world treated women on its head.

Mary Magdalene and the other women, as the first ones to see the risen Messiah, being entrusted with spreading the news of Jesus's resurrection is the most remarkable thing I've ever heard, knowing that their eyewitness testimony generally would not have been legally valid. In a culture that oppressed women into silence and submission, Jesus came to set them free. I love Galatians 3:28 and believe it perfectly summarizes the heart of God for all His people: "There is neither Jew nor Gentile, neither slave nor free, nor is there male and female, for you are all one in Christ Jesus."

Whether we feel hormonal and are running on empty or are thriving and on top of the world, Jesus remains our steady anchor. Through His radical love, women were set free from the chains of society. That freedom shapes the way we think about our embodiment and how we live out our calling. Like Eve, we carry the divine imprint of our Creator—image bearers, helpers, nurturers, and warriors. We are vessels of His Spirit and living testimonies that proclaim His goodness in every season.

THE COST OF CONSTANT DOING

Just as Christ set women free to walk boldly in their calling, He also designed our bodies with an intricate rhythm that speaks of His wisdom and care. Women tend to live in a perpetual state of "go," juggling tasks, meeting deadlines, and managing expectations, all while watching their allostatic load—a fancy term for the cumulative effects chronic stress has on the mind and body—increase. The body wasn't built to sustain prolonged chaos, and the cost of ignoring the big red alarm sounding "Slow down!" is detrimental. Remember point seven from chapter 6? Less is more. The nervous system is always listening for cues, and if the alarm keeps blaring, the body will remain in survival mode.

The nervous system is the body's master communicator. It's like a highway, constantly sending and receiving messages among the brain, organs, muscles, and hormones. It consists of two parts: the central nervous system (CNS), which includes the brain and spinal cord, and the peripheral nervous system (PNS), which includes all the nerves that branch out from the spinal cord. The PNS breaks down further into the autonomic nervous system (ANS), which runs automatic functions like heart rate, breathing, and digestion. The ANS has two branches, the sympathetic (fight or flight) and the parasympathetic (rest and digest). The sympathetic is the body's fear detector, firing the amygdala in response to stress, urgency, pressure, or fear. It pumps adrenaline and cortisol from the adrenal glands, quickens heart rate, tenses muscles, and slows digestion, helping equip you to tackle a scary situation. The sympathetic nervous system is a God-given gift that is needed in some situations, but only in the short term, as we've learned throughout this book. When we get stuck in this system, ignoring the alarm, problems such as hormonal imbalances, anxiety, insomnia, inflammation, and illness can develop.

On the other hand, the parasympathetic is the opposite. It's known as the healing state, activating during relaxation, deep breathing, prayer, sleep, and safety. It slows the heart rate, promotes digestion, supports ovulation, and balances hormones. A key player in the PNS is the vagus nerve, which runs from the brain stem through the neck, chest, heart, and lungs and into the gut. It plays a crucial role in heart rate, digestion, breathing, emotional regulation, and immune response. The strength of the activity in the vagus nerve is called the vagal tone, which can determine how fast or slow one responds to and recovers from stress. A high vagal tone results in faster recovery from stress, a steadier heart rate, better digestion and nutrient absorption, stronger emotional resilience, more balanced hormones, lower inflammation, and more restful sleep. A low vagal tone leads to the opposite.

It's important for women to know where they fall on the scale because chronic stress weakens the vagal tone, which can keep you stuck in fight-or-flight mode and disrupt progesterone levels, cortisol rhythms, and digestion. Especially for those of you who may have no idea where your symptoms are coming from, learning about the state of your nervous system can help point you in the right direction for healing.

Take this brief quiz to explore whether your vagal tone is strong, balanced, or in need of support.

Answer yes or no to each of the following questions:

1. Do you bounce back quickly after stress or conflict?
2. Do you fall asleep easily and stay asleep through the night?
3. Is your digestion generally regular and comfortable?
4. Do you feel emotionally resilient when life is overwhelming?
5. Do you often feel calm and grounded in your body?
6. Do you rarely experience racing thoughts or anxiety?
7. Do you have stable energy throughout the day?
8. Do you recover quickly after physical exertion or illness?
9. Can you take slow, deep breaths without feeling tension?
10. Do you frequently laugh, sing, or connect meaningfully with others?

Reflection

(This is not a diagnosis, only a starting point for self-awareness.)

- **7–10 Yes answers** → You likely have **strong vagal tone** and good parasympathetic regulation.
- **4–6 Yes answers** → You may benefit from more **nervous system support** and stress recovery practices.
- **0–3 Yes answers** → Your vagal tone may be **low**, and your body could be stuck in stress mode.

If you fell in the low vagal tone range, don't panic. Though the nervous system is sensitive, it responds well to change. You're not sentenced to life without parole in the low range! And let us not forget that our God is Jehovah Rapha, our Healer. With Him, all things are possible.

Here are a few exercises you can try to gently strengthen your vagal tone.

- Deep breathing (inhale for four counts, exhale for six to eight)
- Humming, singing, or worshipping (activates the vagus nerve via the vocal cords)
- Cold exposure (splash face with cold water, dunk face in a bowl of ice in the mornings, or try contrast showers)
- Gargling (activates muscles in the throat connected to the vagus nerve)
- Laughter and fruitful connection (safety supports vagal health)
- Gratitude and journaling (grounding techniques)

- Sabbath once a week (self-discipline and forced rest)
- Prayerful stillness (for example, remembering that you are an *ezer* and that God wants to lift your burdens off your shoulders)
- Meditation on Proverbs 31 (meditation and prayer activate the parasympathetic)

Strengthening the vagal tone is more than a nervous system "bio hack"; it's a return to God's design and delight in rest and healing. It's also a reminder that we are strong allies and *ezers* who were created not to carry the weight of life alone but to partner with God and with others. Living as an *ezer* means learning to adapt, not just hyper-fixate on controlling our circumstances. Stressful workdays, nerve-racking presentations, the constant pull of family life—these are unavoidable realities, but God didn't design you to white-knuckle your way through them. Instead, He's given you tools like breath, prayer, movement, joy, and stillness to support your body and spirit so you can show up as the strong helper you were created to be.

Health tip: Emotional tears contain stress hormones like ACTH and cortisol, meaning that crying literally helps your body release built-up tension. That's one reason you often feel calmer, lighter, or sleepy after a good cry.

THE EFFECT OF PRAYER ON YOUR HORMONES

We often think of prayer as something strictly spiritual, but what if I told you it's also biologically impactful? When you pray, your body responds just as much as your spirit. Studies now show what we've intuitively known all along—prayer can calm the mind, soften the body's stress response, and support overall emotional and physiological balance.[4] It's the greatest hormonal reset.

Praying activates the parasympathetic nervous system. You could be physically speaking or singing out loud, sitting in silence, reading or listening to the Word, or breathing while reciting Scripture in your mind. Each of these practices stimulates the vagus nerve, which directly activates the PNS. Your heart rate and blood pressure begin to lower, and your body receives the message *I'm safe.* Just five to ten minutes of slow breathing while praying can shift the body from fight or flight to rest and digest. That's because breath cycles influence different branches of the nervous system.

Inhale → sympathetic → prepares the body for action
Exhale → parasympathetic → calms the body

When you exhale longer than inhale, you tilt your nervous system toward calm and safety. Let's break this down further to fully understand the workmanship of God in our bodies. When the vagus nerve gets stimulated through long exhales, the heart rate slows down, encouraging heart rate variability (HRV), the variation of time between heartbeats—a key marker of vagal tone. A high HRV means your heart can adapt quickly between calm and stress, and a low HRV signals that the response time is delayed, usually indicating chronic stress or nervous system dysfunction. Long exhales also lower cortisol levels and promote relaxation of the chest and diaphragm.

Job 33:4 says, "The Spirit of God has made me; the breath of the Almighty gives me life."

Another way prayer pulls you out of the sympathetic (fight or flight) is through focused attention and stillness. Ever wonder why you can't think rationally when in a moment of panic? When you're flooded with fear, worry, or anxiety, the brain moves all focus away from the prefrontal cortex (processing and decision-making) and sends it to the amygdala (fear center), at the back of the brain. This is why you shouldn't make big life decisions in the heat of the moment! When you pray, that focus returns to the prefrontal cortex, calming the mind, helping you think clearly again. Prayer is the spiritual anchor that keeps us grounded and reminds us that with God, everything will be all right.

Prayer also establishes a sense of safety and trust, two emotions needed for parasympathetic activation. And it's not a solo exercise; it's a relational, intimate conversation with the Father. He listens when you call on Him. First Peter 3:12 assures us of this: "The eyes of the Lord watch over those who do right, and his ears are open to their prayers" (NLT). There's not a moment in prayer or a night spent crying out for help when God isn't listening.

Prayer is a supernatural practice we get to engage in every day. It's more than a one-way conversation. God truly hears and sees you. But He didn't give us prayer only so we could connect with Him; He gave it also to restore us. When you pray, your body slows down, your breath deepens, and stress melts to surrender. In those quiet, holy moments, healing happens: The parasympathetic turns on, prompting peace and a sense of safety throughout your body. And because the body produces reproductive hormones only when it feels safe, prayer tells your body that it doesn't need to stay in survival mode anymore (cortisol) and that it's safe to produce hormones once again (progesterone, estrogen, insulin, etc.).

RETURNING TO HOLY REST

Rest is a sacred, holy practice that the Lord is begging you to take. Jesus says in Matthew 11:28, "Come to me, all you who are weary and burdened, and I will give you rest." The word "weary" in Greek is *kopiaō*—to labor to the point of exhaustion. And "burdened," or *pephortismenoi,* means to be weighed down by carrying heavy loads, like religious pressure, emotional strains, or debilitating menstrual cycles—life stacked on life. But time in prayer with Jesus helps regulate our nervous system. When we're with someone calm, grounded, and safe, our nervous system picks up on those signals, even before we consciously register them. This process is shaped by neuroception, the brain's automatic ability to detect safety or danger in our environment. And this isn't only for those who grew up with a secure lifestyle; this is for the shut-down, never-felt-safe ones who are just now learning what rest means.

It's time to stop measuring your value by your output and start anchoring it in Him who calls you worthy before you even lift a finger. God calls you *ezer*, a helper in the likeness of God, a shield, a strength-bearer and life-giver. But how can you be a shield, one who protects, if you're constantly depleted? Embracing your divine nature is not to grind harder, push through the crippling PMS, or strive further, but rather to live rooted and well rested in Christ. You were made for this holy pause.

So maybe the invitation isn't only to slow down. Maybe it's to *return*.

To the garden.

To your breath.

You were not created to live in survival mode. You were made for still waters, green pastures, unhurried mornings, and peace that surpasses all understanding. The world may glorify the grind, but the Spirit whispers, "Come away with Me."

Slow isn't failure.

Slow is where healing begins.

PRACTICAL APPLICATION

- At the end of the night—regardless of the status of your to-do list—say aloud, "I've done all I could today, and it was more than enough."
- To activate your parasympathetic nervous system, practice exhaling longer than you inhale—inhale for four counts, exhale for six to eight.
- Pick one or two exercises to strengthen your vagal tone.

- Make a de-stress mocktail (see following recipe) to give your nervous system a little extra love (best consumed midmorning or between lunch and dinner).

SCRIPTURE TO MEDITATE ON

- "Come to me, all you who are weary and burdened, and I will give you rest. Take my yoke upon you and learn from me, for I am gentle and humble in heart, and you will find rest for your souls. For my yoke is easy and my burden is light." (Matthew 11:28–30)
- "The eyes of the LORD watch over those who do right, and his ears are open to their prayers." (1 Peter 3:12 NLT)
- "The Spirit of God has made me; the breath of the Almighty gives me life." (Job 33:4)

De-Stress Mocktail

Juice of 1–2 freshly squeezed oranges—for vitamin C

Vitamin C helps regulate the body's stress response by supporting the adrenal glands, the glands responsible for producing cortisol. It also acts as a powerful antioxidant, reducing inflammation.

8 ounces coconut water or filtered water—for magnesium and potassium

Magnesium and potassium are key electrolytes that help calm and stabilize the nervous system, especially when stress has your body feeling tense or depleted. Drinking them helps replenish what stress drains.

2 tablespoons coconut cream—for stabilizing blood sugar

Coconut cream is rich in healthy fats, and fats slow the rate at which glucose is absorbed into the bloodstream. This acts as a balance to the oranges, since orange juice can spike blood sugar quickly.

1 scoop collagen—for bioavailable amino acids

Collagen provides amino acids that help support skin, joints, gut lining, and overall tissue repair, which is especially helpful when under stress.

Pinch of salt, Celtic or Himalayan—for trace minerals

Salt provides essential trace minerals like sodium, magnesium and potassium, that support hydration and healthy nerve function. These minerals help your cells absorb water more effectively.

TWELVE

THE BALANCE OF FAITH AND FEELINGS

I'LL NEVER FORGET HOW IT FELT.

At first it was a racing heart. But then the pins and needles started, like static under my skin. It's never sudden; it's slow and cruel, like quicksand slowly pulling me under. The numbness crept from my feet to my calves, up to my thighs, and into my stomach. Simultaneously my hands clenched and my jaw locked, lips stuck like a wax figure sipping a straw.

I knew the protocol.

Inhale for four, hold for seven, exhale for eight.

That used to work.

Then came the drop—the small, sudden jolt of the plane that made my stomach fall into my legs. A "ding" from the cabin and a flashing light accompanied it. I thought, "That noise surely means we're going down.

The oxygen masks are going to fall any minute." My mind didn't register it as turbulence. No, my nervous system told me a different story.

This is it.

This is the end.

It didn't matter that the other passengers and flight attendants were calm, unbothered by the fact that the plane was clearly about to plummet from the sky; my body was under siege, and no breathing exercise or grounding technique was going to help. I sat there completely immobile, unable to lift my legs, stretch my fingers, or move my mouth. I was paralyzed, desperately crying out to God as tears soaked my shirt. All I could do was recite Psalm 56:3, "When I am afraid, I put my trust in you," over and over until the plane touched ground.

Prayer wasn't enough to give me full mobility back. Fear overrode any hope and peace I felt. When I would catch a moment of calm—a smooth thirty seconds in the air—I'd begin to talk my body out of panic, all for the plane to make another sudden movement and send me right back into paralysis.

That's what a panic attack does: It convinces you that you're not just anxious, you're in danger. It blurs the line between fear and reality until you're no longer sure which one you're in. In moments like that, when your body is screaming and thoughts are spiraling, fear seems to overpower faith. Believe me when I say I know how intense those feelings and emotions can be. I know the power they hold. I know they can convince you of a different reality and trick you into thinking something is true when it's not.

I don't remember how long the panic lasted; time is fuzzy when you're trying to convince yourself you're not about to die. But something lingered long after we landed, a deeper question I had never truly asked myself: What does it mean to be a woman of faith when your emotions feel like tidal waves?

That flight from Los Angeles to New York taught me what no Sunday school class ever did: You can know God is with you and still feel terrified. You can love Jesus with all your heart, soul, and strength and still have a body that betrays you in fear. You can be filled with faith and flooded with feelings all at the same time. And that doesn't make you a "bad" Christian; it makes you human.

From childhood I was made to believe that my emotions and sensitivity were too much, a problem that needed fixing. And since giving my life to Christ, I had associated strong faith with emotional stability (a department I clearly struggle in!). But I've learned that emotions aren't the enemy; they're messengers, showing up to alert you of what's happening inside. They point to fear, worry, pain, and even longing or desire. And while they're real and valid, they're not always true.

Feelings aren't the problem; the problem is believing every feeling as fact.

God never asks us to silence our emotions. In fact, Scripture is full of deeply emotional moments: David weeping in Psalms, Jeremiah grieving in Lamentations, Hannah sobbing in the temple, Jesus sweating blood in the garden of Gethsemane. And they each brought their feelings to God rather than suppressing them and putting them in a box never to be opened. Feelings are healthy and come from the Lord, meaning He feels what we feel, only a million times stronger. Emotions are real, but they're not the ruler. They deserve a seat at the table, just not at the head.

We sometimes unknowingly make our emotions an idol. You may be thinking, "How can I possibly idolize my emotions?" It's simple: Do you follow your feelings more than God? Do you listen to your anxiety more than God? Are you led by fear more than the Lord? Do you act based on how you feel instead of what you know is right? Do you constantly need to "feel" something to validate your faith? The idolization of my feelings was a tough revelation I had when I was twenty-three, fresh out of a breakup. My feelings convinced me there was no hope of a future, and God's whisper of "I have good plans for you" went in one ear and out the other. It's hard to dethrone something you've trusted and found comfort in for so long. But there's only one King who can reign over your life, and He's greater than any temporary emotion or hormone-induced storm.

Throughout this book, we've held space for one another to be fully seen, heard, and loved. We've learned about the anatomy of a woman—how periods work, how the endocrine system operates, and what causes hormonal imbalances and how to help them. We've even cried together while reading stories from women who have walked through heartbreak. But what do we do now? How can we honor our feelings and emotions without letting them drive our faith? When hormones start intensifying our feelings—PMDD, postpartum, etc.—how can we anchor ourselves to Christ? When our body's alarm system won't shut off, how can we pull ourselves out of panic and into peace? How can we create a healthy balance between faith and feelings?

I wish there were a one-size-fits-all answer to these questions. Sometimes it's trial and error, and other times it's a desperate cry to the Lord. I've tried every relaxation technique and read every book but found that nothing worked until I took a hard look in the mirror and admitted that I'm not very kind to myself when I'm not okay. For decades I allowed brutal self-talk to slowly kill me. I dissociated. I gaslit myself into believing I was just being dramatic, difficult, and needy in times when I really just needed a hug. Nobody could have been meaner to me than I was to myself.

Trauma is a confusing, twisted, dark thing. A lot of my issues, and maybe yours too, run so deep it's as if they're hardwired into my DNA. I like to call it "defaulting"—this concept that your brain automatically goes to a certain way of thinking, believing, or behaving. An example of this could be someone canceling plans with you. You default to thinking, "Nobody ever wants to hang out with me. Everyone hates me." Despite the fact that you see this friend often, your brain immediately jumps to negative thoughts. To balance our faith and feelings, we need to work on what we default to. And it takes time, a ton of work, and a whole lot of grace.

Our works can't save us; we are saved by grace through faith. It's this Jesus-wrapped grace that meets us in our default settings, in the emotional tornados sometimes tied to our cycles—the depression that pops up out of nowhere, the emotional highs and lows, and the paralyzing fear. This perfect grace shows up when we feel we're failing ourselves and God. The truth is, faith isn't the absence of feelings; it's the active choice to trust in Him even when our feelings are screaming to do the opposite. It's the willingness to sit with the doubt, grief, or fear and say, "Even here, I believe."

The balance of faith and feelings isn't about becoming emotionally bulletproof. It's learning to discern between the voice of emotions and the voice of the Savior. It's realizing you can love the Lord passionately while wrestling with addiction. You can grieve your chronic medical condition while sobbing into the hem of His garment. You can feel afraid and still be protected. You can feel like your world is falling apart while knowing that God is holding it together.

Grace reminds us that there will be days when the panic wins, when the default patterns return, and when the fear overrides hope, but that doesn't mean God has left us. Slowly, gently, Jesus rewires what we default to. Instead of defaulting to the patterns of the past, we start defaulting to God's truth and promises. Dr. Daniel Amen, a physician and brain health expert, coined the term ANTs (automatic negative thoughts) to describe the "unwanted, unhelpful automatic negative thoughts that get stuck in your mind."[1] The four characteristics of ANTs are that they're rapid and unbidden, negative in nature, emotion-triggering, and based on interpretation.

The nine ANT species are as follows:

1. All-or-Nothing (thinking that things are either all good or all bad)

2. Less-Than (comparing and seeing yourself as less than others)
3. Just-the-Bad (seeing only the bad in a situation)
4. Guilt-Beating (thinking in words like *should, must, have to*)
5. Labeling (attaching a negative label to yourself or others)
6. Fortune-Telling (predicting the worst possible outcome with little or no evidence)
7. Mind-Reading (believing you know what other people are thinking even though they haven't told you)
8. If-Only and I'll-Be-Happy-When (arguing with the past and longing for the future)
9. Blaming (blaming someone else for your problems)

Dr. Amen's tips for killing the ANT infestation are to write down each automatic negative thought as it comes, identify which ANT species it is, then ask yourself if the thought is true. The last step is to ask yourself how you feel when you have the thought and how it would feel *not* to have the thought.

Let's run through a few scenarios together.

Thought: I'm not nearly as pretty as the other women in this room.

ANT species: Less-Than

Is it true? No. I just feel insecure today. I'm four days out from my period, and I feel icky.

How I feel with the thought: I feel even worse.

How I would feel without the thought: I'd feel freer and more confident. I'd be able to enjoy my night and have fun.

Thought: I should be over the breakup by now.

ANT species: Guilt-Beating

Is it true? No. Healing doesn't have a time frame; I know it might take a while.

How I feel with the thought: I feel like I'm falling behind and can't catch up. I feel awful and pathetic for not being able to get over it faster.

How I would feel without the thought: I'd be able to extend grace to myself. The breakup came out of nowhere and shattered my heart, so to think I'm bound to a time frame to heal is unfair. I'd be able to surround myself with godly community and take things one day at a time.

Thought: I'm always going to have painful periods.

ANT species: All-or-Nothing

Is it true? It can be if I don't do anything to try to help myself.

How I feel with the thought: I feel doomed to a bottomless pit of pain with no way out. I'll be stuck forever.

How I would feel without the thought: I would feel like there's hope for pain relief and a possibility for healing. I would feel more in control of my health.

Renewing your mind by changing the type of thoughts you default to is a powerful way to see God's faithfulness in your everyday life and help you balance the war in your brain. Perhaps the best part of following Jesus is that you're never stuck in hopelessness. Your default thoughts *can* be rewired. Neuroplasticity is the brain's ability to change through growth and reorganization. Thank God for that! You're not stuck in your fear. Or doubt. Or grief. Or addiction. And through neuroplasticity, science echoes the truth of Romans 12:2: You can be transformed by the renewing of your mind.

When the world around you and the hormones within you are waging war, anchor yourself to Christ and default to *grace*. Defaulting to grace means that when you mess up, panic, or spiral, you don't shame yourself; you run to Jesus. It means replacing the question "What's wrong with me?" with "What does God say about me?" It's pausing in the middle of the crying, the cramps, the screaming baby, the loss and asking God to remind you who you are. You won't always *feel* His presence, but faith isn't about what you feel; it's about who you trust.

Faith says, "Even when I don't feel it, I believe You're here. Even when my body is in panic mode, I trust that You're in control. Even when I can't see a way out, I believe You'll show me the way." And slowly, belief becomes your baseline. God does something profound in the wrestling between truth and tenderness, hope and honesty, worship and weeping. You don't have to fake peace to prove faith. You just have to let Jesus meet you in your reality, because you were never meant to choose between being holy and hormonal. You were made to be both—holy in your spirit, hormonal in your humanity, and held together by a God who honors it all.

ACKNOWLEDGMENTS

FIRST AND FOREMOST, I WOULDN'T BE HERE WITHOUT THE GOOD-ness and faithfulness of my Lord and Savior, Jesus Christ. He pulled me out of the pit and placed my feet on solid ground. Without His love and grace, I am nothing. This book was His idea, and it's the honor of a lifetime that He entrusted me to steward it. All that I am is because of God, and He gets all the glory.

To my parents for their unwavering support throughout my life. My mom has modeled what being a confident, go-getter woman looks like and has selflessly given me all I've ever needed and wanted day in and day out. Without her I wouldn't be the woman I am today. Mom, you inspire me, and I love you to pieces. To my dad for loving me unconditionally and showing me what being a safe space means. You answer every phone call—sometimes multiple times a day—and never fail to send the nicest texts throughout the week to remind me how much you love me. You both have never left my side through all the trials, hospital visits, checkups, and hormonal ups and downs—you guys are my heroes.

To my husband, Frank, for happily taking the baton from my parents and saying yes to forever with me. You're my rock, my better half, the one who encourages me when I feel like I can't go any further, and the one I laugh with until I can't breathe. Life with you is a dream. Jesus really outdid Himself when He gave me you. There aren't enough words to describe my love for you.

To my agent, Kathleen, at Alive Literary Agency for fully jumping on board the second I told her about my idea for a book about Jesus and periods. Never once did you doubt me, this ministry, or my career as an author. Thank you for being my biggest cheerleader.

To my editor, Andrea, at Zondervan for eagerly taking me under your wing and being my greatest advocate. You've graciously walked with me through the entire publishing process, always lifting me up when I felt like I wasn't good enough to write this book. Your support is what got me through the long nights. I'm beyond grateful for you and the entire Zondervan team.

To the women who have followed my journey on social media over the years: You are what keeps me going. Reading your messages of encouragement and listening to your personal stories about your hormones make all the hard work worth it. You are my hype girls, and I can always count on you. I hope you feel the love reciprocated.

To all the women who shared their stories of loss, grief, miscarriage, and the many complexities of womanhood: Thank you for being so brave and for entrusting me with your journeys.

And lastly, to you, reader: Thank you for your curiosity, desire to learn, and willingness to grow. I had you in mind every time I sat down to write these chapters. Know that you are never alone in your battle—you have a sister in me always. I pray that the Lord wraps His loving arms around you as He continues writing your story.

GLOSSARY

adrenal fatigue—A nonmedical term describing the exhaustion of the adrenal glands after prolonged stress, leaving the body unable to cope well.

adrenal glands—Small glands above the kidneys that produce stress hormones like cortisol and adrenaline. They are vital for energy, resilience, and responsiveness to life's demands.

adrenaline (epinephrine)—A stress hormone released during a fight-or-flight response that increases heart rate and alertness.

allopregnanolone—A calming brain chemical made from progesterone that supports mood balance and reduces anxiety.

amenorrhea—The absence of menstruation, often linked to stress, hormonal imbalance, or underlying conditions.

amygdala—A part of the brain that processes emotions like fear, stress, and anxiety.

androgens—A group of hormones (including testosterone) that regulates sexual development, energy, and muscle mass.

anovulation—A cycle where ovulation does not occur, common in PCOS or under high stress.

aromatization—The process of converting androgens (like testosterone) into estrogen.

autoimmunity—When the immune system mistakenly attacks the body's own tissues.

autonomic nervous system—The automatic control system regulating heart rate, digestion, breathing, and stress response.

basal body temperature (BBT)—The body's lowest temperature at rest, often tracked to identify ovulation patterns.

bioavailability—How well the body absorbs and uses a nutrient or medication.

bioindividuality—The principle that each person's body and health needs are unique.

birth control—Medications or devices used to prevent pregnancy by altering hormones or blocking conception.

bloating—A common menstrual symptom caused by hormonal shifts or fluid retention, reminding us that the body speaks through discomfort.

blood sugar regulation—The balance of glucose in the blood, key for energy, mood, and hormone stability.

cervical mucus—The fluid produced by the cervix that changes throughout the cycle, acting as a fertility sign.

circadian rhythm—The body's internal twenty-four-hour clock that regulates sleep, energy, and hormone release.

cortisol—The main stress hormone, essential for survival but harmful when chronically elevated.

cycle syncing—Aligning lifestyle, nutrition, and activity with the phases of the menstrual cycle to work *with* the body rather than against it.

DHEA (dehydroepiandrosterone)—A hormone made by the adrenal glands that helps produce estrogen and testosterone.

dopamine—A neurotransmitter tied to motivation, reward, and pleasure, reminding us of God's design for joy and fulfillment.

dysmenorrhea—Painful menstrual cramps.

endocrine system—The network of glands (thyroid, adrenals, ovaries, etc.) that releases hormones to regulate the body's balance.

endometriosis—A painful condition where uterine-like tissue grows outside the uterus, often delaying diagnosis for women.

estrobolome—The collection of gut bacteria that helps regulate estrogen metabolism.

estrogen—A primary female hormone that supports fertility, bone health, mood, and cardiovascular health.

estrogen dominance—A state where estrogen levels are high relative to progesterone, often causing PMS, heavy periods, and mood changes.

ezer—A Hebrew word used in Scripture for "helper," describing women as strong allies, protectors, and life-givers reflecting God's own nature.

fallopian tubes—The tubes connecting the ovaries to the uterus, where fertilization occurs.

fertility window—The days in the menstrual cycle when conception is most likely, designed with precision by God.

follicle—A small fluid-filled sac in the ovary that holds an immature egg until ovulation.

follicular phase—The first half of the menstrual cycle after menstruation, when estrogen rises and the body prepares for ovulation.

free radicals—Unstable molecules that damage cells, often countered by antioxidants.

FSH (follicle-stimulating hormone)—A hormone that stimulates ovarian follicles to grow and mature before ovulation.

functional medicine—An approach that looks at root causes of health issues, not only symptoms.

GABA (gamma-aminobutyric acid)—A calming neurotransmitter that helps reduce stress and anxiety; God's built-in peace regulator.

ghrelin—The "hunger hormone" that stimulates appetite.

glucagon—A hormone released by the pancreas that raises blood sugar by signaling the liver to release stored glucose.

glucose—The body's main energy source, derived from carbohydrates.

GnRH (gonadotropin-releasing hormone)—A hormone released by the brain that signals the ovaries to produce estrogen and progesterone.

gut microbiome—The trillions of bacteria in the digestive tract that influence health and hormones.

homeostasis—The body's natural balance maintained by hormones and systems working together.

hormone—A chemical messenger made by glands in the endocrine system that travels through the bloodstream to regulate processes such as mood, energy, fertility, growth, and metabolism. Hormones act like signals that tell your body when to start, stop, or adjust specific functions, keeping everything in balance.

HPA axis (hypothalamic-pituitary-adrenal axis)—The communication system between the brain and adrenal glands that regulates stress response.

hypothalamus—A brain region that acts as the master regulator of hormones, sleep, and appetite.

hypothyroidism—A condition where the thyroid is underactive, slowing metabolism.

inflammation—The body's immune response that can become chronic, impacting hormones and menstrual health.

infradian rhythm—A biological rhythm that lasts longer than twenty-four hours, such as the menstrual cycle.

insulin—The hormone that regulates blood sugar, essential for energy but harmful when resistance develops.

insulin resistance—A condition where the body doesn't respond properly to insulin, often linked to PCOS and metabolic issues.

integrative medicine—An approach combining conventional medicine with holistic therapies for whole-body healing.

leptin—A hormone that signals satiety and helps regulate metabolism.

LH (luteinizing hormone)—The hormone that triggers ovulation.

libido—Sexual drive, influenced by hormones like testosterone.

luteal phase—The second half of the menstrual cycle, marked by progesterone dominance and often PMS symptoms.

magnesium—A mineral crucial for hormone balance, sleep, and stress support, often called the "relaxation mineral."

melatonin—The hormone that regulates sleep and circadian rhythms.

menopause—The natural end of the menstrual cycle; a new season of womanhood still designed with purpose by God.

menstrual cycle—The monthly hormonal rhythm preparing the body for pregnancy.

menstrual phase—The first phase of the menstrual cycle, marked by bleeding as the uterine lining sheds.

menstruation—The shedding of the uterine lining, a monthly rhythm that reflects both renewal and rest.

metabolism—The process by which your body converts food into energy, supporting growth, repair, and daily function.

microbiome—The collection of bacteria and microbes in the gut that influences immunity and hormones.

micronutrients—Essential vitamins and minerals required for hormone health.

neuroplasticity—The brain's ability to rewire and adapt over time.

neurotransmitters—Chemical messengers that carry signals between brain and body, regulating mood, sleep, and stress.

omega-3 fatty acids—Anti-inflammatory fats that support hormones, fertility, and brain function.

ovarian cysts—Fluid-filled sacs that form on the ovaries, common in hormonal imbalance like PCOS.

ovaries—Female glands that produce eggs, estrogen, and progesterone.

ovulation—The release of an egg from the ovary, a central event of the menstrual cycle.

ovulatory phase—The phase when the egg is released from the ovary, around midcycle.

oxytocin—The "love hormone" released during intimacy, childbirth, and breastfeeding that fosters bonding.

pancreas—The gland that produces insulin and regulates blood sugar.

parabens—Synthetic preservatives found in cosmetics and personal care products, known to be endocrine disruptors.

parasympathetic nervous system—The "rest and digest" system that calms the body after stress.

PCOS (polycystic ovary syndrome)—A hormonal disorder that affects ovulation, insulin sensitivity, and fertility.

perimenopause—The years leading up to menopause when a woman's cycle shifts and hormone fluctuations intensify.

period—Another term for menstruation, the shedding of the uterine lining.

phthalates—Chemicals in plastics and fragrances that disrupt hormones and affect reproductive health.

pituitary gland—The "master gland" that regulates many hormones.

PMDD (premenstrual dysphoric disorder)—A severe form of PMS with mood and physical symptoms.

PMS (premenstrual syndrome)—Physical and emotional symptoms before menstruation.

pregnenolone—A precursor hormone from which cortisol, progesterone, and estrogen are made.

pregnenolone steal—A phenomenon in which the body, in response to chronic stress, diverts pregnenolone (a precursor hormone) away from making sex hormones like progesterone, estrogen, and testosterone and instead uses it to produce more cortisol.

progesterone—A hormone crucial for calming the body, supporting pregnancy, and balancing estrogen.

prostaglandins—Compounds that cause uterine contractions, often linked to painful periods.

serotonin—The "feel good" neurotransmitter tied to mood and happiness.

sperm—Male reproductive cells that fertilize the female egg.

spiritual warfare—The unseen battle between God's kingdom and the Enemy, often heightened when women feel weak or vulnerable.

stress—A natural response that becomes damaging when chronic, impacting hormones deeply.

supplements—Concentrated sources of nutrients, herbs, or compounds used to support health.

sympathetic nervous system—The fight-or-flight system activated by stress.

testosterone—An androgen important for energy, libido, and muscle mass, present in both men and women.

thyroid—A butterfly-shaped gland in the neck that regulates metabolism and energy.

thyroid hormones (T3, T4)—Hormones that control metabolism and growth.

uterus—The womb: the part of the body where a baby grows. It's located slightly below the belly button.

vagal tone—The strength of vagus nerve activity, influencing stress resilience.

vagus nerve—The longest cranial nerve, linking brain and body, regulating rest, digestion, and resilience.

vitamins—Essential organic compounds the body needs in small amounts to function properly.

xenoestrogens—Chemicals from plastics, pesticides, and beauty products that mimic estrogen and disrupt hormonal balance.

NOTES

INTRODUCTION

1. "History of Women's Participation in Clinical Research," NIH Inclusion Outreach Toolkit: How to Engage, Recruit, and Retain Women in Clinical Research, Office of Research on Women's Health, National Institutes of Health, April 24, 2024, https://orwh.od.nih.gov/toolkit/recruitment/history.
2. Jecca R. Steinberg, Brannon T. Weeks, Griselda A. Reyes, et al., "The Obstetrical Research Landscape: A Cross-Sectional Analysis of Clinical Trials from 2007–2020," *American Journal of Obstetrics and Gynecology MFM* 3, no. 1 (January 2021): 100253, https://www.doi.org/10.1016/j.ajogmf.2020.100253.
3. Jennifer R. Southall, "Disparities Persist in Clinical Trial Leadership Across Specialties," Women in Oncology, Healio, October 30, 2023, https://www.healio.com/news/hematology-oncology/20231030/disparities-persist-in-clinical-trial-leadership-across-specialties.

CHAPTER 1: IT'S NOT YOUR FAULT YOU DIDN'T KNOW

1. "About the Untreated Syphilis Study at Tuskegee," Centers for Disease Control and Prevention, September 4, 2024, https://www.cdc.gov/tuskegee/about/index.html.
2. Alyson J. McGregor, "Medical Research Has Left Women in the Dark for Years. Here's How We Change It," Katz Institute for Women's Health, Northwell Health, accessed October 27, 2025, www.northwell.edu/katz-institute-for-womens-health/articles/medical-research.

3. McGregor, "Medical Research Has Left Women in the Dark for Years. Here's How We Change It."
4. "Endometriosis: Defining It, Recognizing It, and Treating It," Endometriosis Foundation of America, September 28, 2022, https://www.endofound.org/endometriosis.
5. Melanie Gibson-Helm, Helena Teede, Andrea Dunaif, and Anuja Dokras, "Delayed Diagnosis and a Lack of Information Associated with Dissatisfaction in Women with Polycystic Ovary Syndrome," *Journal of Clinical Endocrinology and Metabolism* 102, no. 2 (February 2017): 604–12, https://doi.org/10.1210/jc.2016-2963.
6. Sohyeon Kwon, Rockli Kim, Jong-Tae Lee, et al., "Association of Smartphone Use with Body Image Distortion and Weight Loss Behaviors in Korean Adolescents," *JAMA Network Open* 5, no. 5 (2022): e2213237, https://doi.org/10.1001/jamanetworkopen.2022.13237.

CHAPTER 2: THE FOUR SEASONS OF YOUR CYCLE

1. "Menstruation in Girls and Adolescents: Using the Menstrual Cycle as a Vital Sign," ACOG, December 2015, https://www.acog.org/clinical/clinical-guidance/committee-opinion/articles/2015/12/menstruation-in-girls-and-adolescents-using-the-menstrual-cycle-as-a-vital-sign.
2. "Period Irregularities to Get Checked Out," Mayo Clinic, April 22, 2023, https://www.mayoclinic.org/healthy-lifestyle/womens-health/in-depth/menstrual-cycle/art-20047186.
3. "Menstruation in Girls and Adolescents," https://www.acog.org/clinical/clinical-guidance/committee-opinion/articles/2015/12/menstruation-in-girls-and-adolescents-using-the-menstrual-cycle-as-a-vital-sign.

CHAPTER 3: YOU'RE NOT CRAZY, YOUR HORMONES ARE IMBALANCED

1. "11 Unexpected Signs of Hormonal Imbalance," Northwell Health, November 27, 2018, https://www.northwell.edu/obstetrics-and-gynecology/fertility/expert-insights/11-unexpected-signs-of-hormonal-imbalance.

2. Alisa Vitti, *WomanCode: Perfect Your Cycle, Amplify Your Fertility, Supercharge Your Sex Drive, and Become a Power Source* (HarperOne, 2013).
3. "Infertility: Frequently Asked Questions," Centers for Disease Control and Prevention: Reproductive Health, May 15, 2024, www.cdc.gov/reproductive-health/infertility-faq/index.html
4. "The Impact of Sleep on Appetite and Metabolism," Mount Sinai, November 27, 2012, https://health.mountsinai.org/blog/the-impact-of-sleep-on-appetite-and-metabolism/.
5. "Nearly 1.8 Billion Adults at Risk of Disease from Not Doing Enough Physical Activity," World Health Organization, June 26, 2024, https://www.who.int/news/item/26-06-2024-nearly-1.8-billion-adults-at-risk-of-disease-from-not-doing-enough-physical-activity.
6. "Infertility: Frequently Asked Questions."
7. R. S. Rivlin, "Magnesium Deficiency and Alcohol Intake: Mechanisms, Clinical Significance and Possible Relation to Cancer Development (A Review)," *Journal of the American College of Nutrition* 13, no. 5 (October 1994): 416–23, https://doi.org/10.1080/07315724.1994.10718430.
8. María del Mar Fernández, Jurgita Saulyte, Hazel M. Inskip, and Bahi Takkouche, "Premenstrual Syndrome and Alcohol Consumption: A Systematic Review and Meta-Analysis," *BMJ Open* 8, no. 3 (April 16, 2018): https://doi.org/10.1136/bmjopen-2017-019490.
9. "Epigenetics, Health, and Disease," Centers for Disease Control and Prevention, January 31, 2025, www.cdc.gov/genomics-and-health/epigenetics/index.html.
10. "How to Increase Estrogen Naturally," UCLA Health, June 2, 2023, www.uclahealth.org/news/article/how-increase-estrogen-naturally.
11. Stepan Feduniw, Lidia Korczyńska, Konrad Górski, et al., "The Effect of Vitamin E Supplementation in Postmenopausal Women—A Systematic Review," *Nutrients* 15, no. 1 (December 2022), article 160, https://www.doi.org/10.3390/nu15010160.

12. "The Pg/E2 (Progesterone/Estradiol) Ratio - ZRT Laboratory," ZRT Laboratory, March 31, 2015, https://www.zrtlab.com/blog/archive/progesterone-estradiol-pg-e2-ratio/.
13. Korey DiRoma, "How to Support Estrogen Detoxification Naturally," Stram Center for Integrative Medicine, April 3, 2025, stramcenter.com/blog/blog-detail/how-to-support-estrogen-detoxification-naturally.
14. University of Michigan, "Feeling Close to a Friend Increases Progesterone, Boosts Well-Being and Reduces Anxiety and Stress," ScienceDaily, June 3, 2009, www.sciencedaily.com/releases/2009/06/090602171941.htm.
15. "Premenstrual Dysphoric Disorder (PMDD)," Johns Hopkins Medicine, accessed October 29, 2025, www.hopkinsmedicine.org/health/conditions-and-diseases/premenstrual-dysphoric-disorder-pmdd.
16. Liisa Hantsoo and Jennifer L. Payne, "Towards Understanding the Biology of Premenstrual Dysphoric Disorder: From Genes to GABA," *Neuroscience and Biobehavioral Reviews* 149 (June 2023), https://www.doi.org/10.1016/j.neubiorev.2023.105168.
17. Jayashri Kulkarni et al., "The Prevalence of Early Life Trauma in Premenstrual Dysphoric Disorder (PMDD)," *Psychiatry Research* 308 (February 2022), article 114381, https://www.doi.org/10.1016/j.psychres.2021.114381.
18. "Polycystic Ovary Syndrome," World Health Organization, February 7, 2025, https://www.who.int/news-room/fact-sheets/detail/polycystic-ovary-syndrome.
19. John C. Marshall and Andrea Dunaif, "Should All Women with PCOS Be Treated for Insulin Resistance?," *Fertility and Sterility* 97, no. 1 (December 19, 2011): 18–22, https://doi.org/10.1016/j.fertnstert.2011.11.036.
20. Jolene Brighten, "Treating PCOS Symptoms: With or Without the Pill," Dr. Jolene Brighten, October 4, 2024, https://drbrighten.com/treating-pcos-symptoms-with-the-pill-or-even-better-without/.
21. Jolene Brighten, "How to Lose Weight With PCOS," Dr.

Jolene Brighten, October 3, 2024, https://drbrighten.com/how-to-lose-weight-with-pcos/.

22. Jacob P. Christ and Marcelle I. Cedars, "Current Guidelines for Diagnosing PCOS," *Diagnostics* 13, no. 6 (March 15, 2023): 1113, https://doi.org/10.3390/diagnostics13061113.
23. Kimberly Daniels and Joyce C. Abma, "Current Contraceptive Status Among Women Aged 15–49: United States, 2015–2017," NCHS Data Brief no. 327, National Center for Health Statistics, December 2018, www.cdc.gov/nchs/products/databriefs/db327.htm.
24. Jolene Brighten, "Period Gone Missing After the Pill? Here's What to Do First," Dr. Brighten, October 11, 2024, drbrighten.com/period-gone-missing-birth-control-pill/.
25. M. Palmery, A. Saraceno, A. Vaiarelli, and G. Carlomagno, "Oral Contraceptives and Changes in Nutritional Requirements," *European Review for Medical and Pharmacological Sciences* 17, no. 13 (July 2013): 1804–13, pubmed.ncbi.nlm.nih.gov/23852908.
26. Monique Tello, "Can Hormonal Birth Control Trigger Depression?," Harvard Health Publishing, October 1, 2019, www.health.harvard.edu/blog/can-hormonal-birth-control-trigger-depression-201610172517.

CHAPTER 6: TEN THINGS EVERY WOMAN SHOULD KNOW ABOUT HER HORMONES

1. John S. White, "Straight Talk About High-Fructose Corn Syrup: What It Is and What It Ain't," *American Journal of Clinical Nutrition* 88, no. 6 (December 2008): 1716S–1721S, https://doi.org/10.3945/ajcn.2008.25825B.
2. Karolina Nowak et al., "Parabens and Their Effects on the Endocrine System," *Molecular and Cellular Endocrinology* 474 (March 26, 2018): 238–51, https://doi.org/10.1016/j.mce.2018.03.014.
3. William R. Lovallo et al., "Cortisol Responses to Mental Stress, Exercise, and Meals Following Caffeine Intake in Men and Women," *Pharmacology Biochemistry and Behavior* 83, no. 3 (May 2, 2006): 441–47, https://doi.org/10.1016

/j.pbb.2006.03.005; Maggie Fox, "Study Links Caffeine with Pregnancy Loss," NBC News, March 24, 2016, www.nbcnews.com/health/womens-health/study-links -caffeine-pregnancy-loss-n544856.

4. Yvonne Chu, "How Sleep Affects Your Immune System," Yale Medicine, March 13, 2023, www.yalemedicine.org /news/how-sleep-affects-immunity.
5. "Aromatization," ScienceDirect, accessed October 30, 2025, www.sciencedirect.com/topics/nursing-and-health -professions/aromatization.

CHAPTER 7: YOUR BODY IS A TEMPLE. SERIOUSLY.

1. "What Were the Holy Place and the Most Holy Place in the Temple/Tabernacle?" GotQuestions.org, January 4, 2022, www.gotquestions.org/Most-Holy-Place.html.

CHAPTER 9: A BIBLICAL APPROACH TO CYCLE SYNCING

1. "The Cycle Syncing Method," accessed October 30, 2025, www.cycle-syncing.com.
2. Selma P. Wiertsema et al., "The Interplay Between the Gut Microbiome and the Immune System in the Context of Infectious Diseases Throughout Life and the Role of Nutrition in Optimizing Treatment Strategies," *Nutrients* 13, no. 3 (2021), article 886, https://doi.org/10.3390/nu13030886.
3. Diane Quagliani and Patricia Felt-Gunderson, "Closing America's Fiber Intake Gap: Communication Strategies from a Food and Fiber Summit," *American Journal of Lifestyle Medicine* 11, no. 1 (July 2016): 80–85, https://doi.org /10.1177/1559827615588079.
4. "Millions of Americans are Vitamin D Deficient—Who Is Most at Risk?," GrassrootsHealth, August 12, 2025, https:// www.grassrootshealth.net/blog/millions-of-americans -are-vitamin-d-deficient-who-is-most-at-risk/.
5. Linda L. Demer, Jeffrey J. Hsu, and Yin Tintut, et al., "Steroid Hormone Vitamin D: Implications for Cardiovascular Disease," *Circulation Research* 122, no. 11 (May 2018): 39–45, https://doi.org/10.1161/CIRCRESAHA.118.311585.

6. Mohammad Mehdi Mohammadi et al., "Effect of Omega-3 Fatty Acids on Premenstrual Syndrome: A Systematic Review and Meta-Analysis," *Journal of Obstetrics and Gynaecology Research* 48, no. 6 (March 9, 2022): 1293–1305, https://doi.org/10.1111/jog.15217.
7. Sanjay Basak, Rahul Mallick, and Asim K. Duttaroy, "Maternal Docosahexaenoic Acid Status During Pregnancy and Its Impact on Infant Neurodevelopment," *Nutrients* 12, no. 12 (2020), article 3615, https://doi.org/10.3390/nu12123615.
8. Abeba Haile Mariamenatu and Emebet Mohammed Abdu, "Overconsumption of Omega-6 Polyunsaturated Fatty Acids (PUFAs) Versus Deficiency of Omega-3 PUFAs in Modern-Day Diets: The Disturbing Factor for Their 'Balanced Antagonistic Metabolic Functions' in the Human Body," *Journal of Lipids* 2021 (March 17, 2021): 1–15, https://doi.org/10.1155/2021/8848161.
9. "Do Women Need to Take Magnesium? Here's the Experts' Verdict," Lucy Notarantonio, Newsweek, November 2, 2024, https://www.newsweek.com/do-women-need-take-magnesium-expert-verdict-1978440.
10. Uwe Gröber, Joachim Schmidt, and Klaus Kisters, "Magnesium in Prevention and Therapy," *Nutrients* 7, no. 9 (September 23, 2015): 8199–8226, https://doi.org/10.3390/nu7095388.

CHAPTER 10: STORE YOUR OIL

1. Cleveland Clinic, "Is Earthing Actually Good for You? Here's What We Know," Cleveland Clinic, April 19, 2024, https://health.clevelandclinic.org/earthing.

CHAPTER 11: SLOW IS STILL HOLY

1. @iamjuliesantiago, "Instagram," October 12, 2025, https://www.instagram.com/iamjuliesantiago/p/DPtqGgBDRih/.
2. Anna Medaris, "Women Say They're Stressed, Misunderstood, and Alone," American Psychological Association, November 1, 2023, www.apa.org/topics/stress/women-stress.

3. Sue Bohlin, "Christianity: The Best Thing That Ever Happened to Women," Bible.org, March 16, 2010, https://bible.org/article/christianity-best-thing-ever-happened-women.
4. Matej Bělousov, "The Influence of Private Christian Prayer Types on Mental and Physical Health," *Proceedings of the MEi:CogSci Conference* 19, no. 1 (2025), https://journals.phl.univie.ac.at/meicogsci/article/view/1007.

CHAPTER 12: THE BALANCE OF FAITH AND FEELINGS

1. "Automatic Negative Thoughts (ANTs): How to Stop Toxic Thinking and Rewire Your Brain," Amen Clinics, June 4, 2025, www.amenclinics.com/blog/negative-thinking-do-you-have-an-ant-infestation-in-your-head/.